GETTING IN

T0237254

GETTING IN

PAUL JUNG

How NOT to Apply to Medical School

Sage Publications, Inc.
International Educational and Professional Publisher
Thousand Oaks ■ London ■ New Delhi

Copyright © 2000 by Sage Publications, Inc.

All rights reserved. No part of this book may be reproduced or utilized in any form or by any means, electronic or mechanical, including photocopying, recording, or by any information storage and retrieval system, without permission in writing from the publisher.

For information:

Sage Publications, Inc.
2455 Teller Road
Thousand Oaks, California 91320
E-mail: order@sagepub.com

Sage Publications Ltd.
6 Bonhill Street
London EC2A 4PU
United Kingdom

Sage Publications India Pvt. Ltd.
M-32 Market
Greater Kailash I
New Delhi 110 048 India

Printed in the United States of America

Library of Congress Cataloging-in-Publication Data

Jung, Paul, 1969-
    Getting in: How *not* to apply to medical school / by Paul Jung.
        p. cm. — (Surviving medical school)
    Includes index.
    ISBN 0-7619-1757-8
    1. Medical colleges—United States—Admission. 2. Medical colleges—United States—Entrance requirements. I. Title.
II. Series.
    R838.4.J85   1999
    610′.71′173—dc21   99-6519

This book is printed on acid-free paper.

00 01 02 03 04 10 9 8 7 6 5 4 3 2 1

Acquiring Editor: Jim Nageotte
Editorial Assistant: Heidi Van Middlesworth
Production Editor: Wendy Westgate
Editorial Assistant: Nevair Kabakian
Copy Editor: Linda Gray
Designer/Typesetter: Janelle LeMaster
Cover Designer: Ravi Balasuriya

Contents

To Dru Bagwell and Nancy Love for all their
valuable advice and guidance.

Foreword

There are more applicants to medical school than ever before—about 57,000 in a recent year—and competition is rough. Although most students have a fundamental understanding of the admissions process, most lack the savvy that will give them an advantage. True, good grades and high MCAT (Medical College Admission Test) scores are important, but when there are so many applicants with sterling academic records, they may not be good enough.

Most premed students spend an inordinate amount of time trying to increase these numerical markers and not enough time taking advantage of opportunities that will set themselves apart from the crowd. This book, providing you with the insight you will need to do this, will enhance your admissions opportunities.

Premed students advised by the author, Paul Jung, M.D., have had a remarkably high medical school acceptance rate. An internal medicine resident at Case Western Reserve University's MetroHealth Medical Center, Dr. Jung is Director of the Health Policy Leadership Institute. In addition to health policy work with Citizen Action, he served as a member of the Clinton Administration Health Care Reform Task Force, worked in San Francisco and Los Angeles on the California Proposition 186 campaign, and was Legislative Affairs Director for the American Medical Student Association. The 1998 recipient of the Fitzhugh Mullan, M.D. Award for Outstanding Resident Physician Leadership, Dr. Jung has served on the boards of Physicians for a National Health Program, the American Medical Student Association, and the Asian Pacific American Medical Student Association.

If you want to avoid common mistakes that may diminish your chance for admission, read this book carefully and implement Dr. Jung's recommendations.

—Robert Holman Coombs
Professor of Behavioral Sciences, UCLA School of Medicine
Series Editor

Acknowledgments

This book could not have been completed without the wise guidance of my early mentors who provided much of the advice I've put on these pages. Special thanks to Dru Bagwell and Nancy Love, as well as my wife, Helen, who has always encouraged me to think differently.

Introduction

When I began college, I knew I wanted to be a doctor. So I did what all my premed friends did: majored in biology, signed up for extra science courses, and became active in the school's premedical society. But after awhile, I started to wonder if I was doing the right thing.

Mostly, I felt as if I was missing out on the college experience and, more important, on a good college education. Luckily, I had one of the best premedical advisers around. She took me aside and told me to go ahead and major in philosophy, stop working in a lab, give up my volunteer time at the local hospital, and write the great American novel instead.

This book isn't exactly the great American novel, but it's an outgrowth of what I learned from that crucial conversation. What she was trying to tell me was that I should pursue my own unique individuality, seriously develop some nonmedical interests, and do what comes naturally. Not only would I be much happier, I might have a better chance of getting into medical school.

She was right. You probably don't care that I had a great time in college, but not only did I get into several medical schools, I was admitted early in the application cycle without a problem and simply had to spend most of my time trying to figure out which school to attend.

The irony is, many of my premed friends did not get into medical school. So I developed these strategies for other students, spent some time as a student premedical adviser myself, and finally created my own medical school admissions consulting service.

These strategies work. They're time-tested and backed up with solid data. Read on.

Why Read This Book?

There are more applicants to medical school than ever before—well over 50,000 applicants in 1998 alone. And these applicants are fighting for a mere 16,000 seats. Competition is rough. Most students have a fundamental understanding of the admission process, but they seriously lack the real savvy that will give them the extra edge in medical school admissions.

There are numerous books on the market that try to tell you how to get into medical school. However, many of them are simply catalogs listing each medical school, along with the positive and negative aspects of each; their titles should instead read, "Ways to Compare Medical Schools." Most admissions advice is dry and plain and tends to simply state the facts about applying without providing any savvy on applying *well.*

Good grades and high MCAT (Medical College Admission Test) scores are great, but they're never good enough, especially with so many applicants these days. Most students spend an inordinate amount of time simply trying to up those numeric values and not enough time taking advantage of the numerous opportunities within the application process to set themselves apart from the crowd.

Other books also tend to concentrate on the regular process of applying to medical school, but they ignore the special circumstances of individual applicants. They also ignore, and thus encourage, applicants to make common mistakes. By taking an alternative spin, this book will allow readers to not simply apply to medical school but to avoid common mistakes and thus apply properly to medical school.

This book will provide applicants with the savvy to use those opportunities and not to miss out. By using the techniques in this book (i.e., by avoiding common mistakes), applicants will have a better chance of getting admitted to medical school in general and also into their medical school of choice.

Many chapters have a vignette called "Egregious Error" that discusses how common, severe mistakes are made by many medical school applicants. These mistakes were made by real students who later came to me for (proper) advice.

Who Should Read This Book?

The primary reader of this book will be the premed student, typically a college sophomore and junior. But this book also has pertinent sections designed for the diligent student who begins thinking about applying early on—say, a freshman or sophomore, even a high school student. Also, this book has significant advice for postbaccalaureate students, those who've spent time after college in the real world, even those who are looking for a more fulfilling second career. This segment of the applicant pool is increasing and demands unique advice. And finally, many college premedical advisers should use this book to illustrate to their students the common mistakes made by many applicants.

PUBLISHER'S NOTE: To the best of our knowledge, mailing addresses, phone numbers, e-mail addresses, and Website addresses are correct, but this information—especially Website addresses, e-mail addresses, and telephone area codes—may change over time.

Section I
Preparation Is Everything

It's never too early to begin applying to medical school. I tell people that the ninth grade is the best place to start, if not earlier, but most people seek my advice after they've already started college, some after they've been rejected from medical school once. Most of the advice in this book will be geared toward students who are still relatively early in their undergraduate college years. Of note, there is a special section for postbaccalaureate students in Chapter 6.

Here I'll begin by presenting a distilled version of this book in the following list:

Ten Easy Ways NOT To Get Into Medical School

  10. Major in biology

   9. Volunteer in a hospital

   8. Work in a lab

   7. Take more science classes

   6. Take the September MCAT again and again

   5. Apply just before the deadline

   4. Apply to identical schools

   3. Apply early decision

   2. Get only three recommendation letters

   1. Write *For Whom the Bell Tolls*

Can't believe what you're reading? The list definitely strays from the standard advice that most premed students receive. Obviously, it's not as simple as the list implies, but there is a large nugget of truth in the statements above. As you read on, you'll understand that the items in the above list are simply indicators of an unsuccessful applicant's herd mentality and ignorance of unique individuality.

1 First Principles

The overriding theme in this book is the development of your unique individuality. Sure, it sounds like some New Age trend like crystals or herbs, but it's just a term I use to identify the traits that separate successful applicants from unsuccessful ones.

Promote Your Unique Individuality

What separates you from the pack? What makes you different from all the other premed students you've met? What distinguishes you from the other 56,000 medical school applicants?

In short, what is your unique individuality? This is the question you should be asking yourself throughout your application process. The answer to this question is what you need to emphasize in your application to get yourself noticed and to get yourself into medical school.

From years of experience, I've noticed two types of applications to medical school: the "standard" application and the "unique" application. The standard application simply relates how well the applicant has followed the herd by majoring in biology, volunteering in a hospital, and working in a lab. Basically, this application is typical, usual, and undistinguished. Those who submit applications of this type are competing with tens of thousands of other applicants who have identical applications. Imagine a roulette wheel with identical colors on it. Instead, the unique application promotes the applicant's individuality and highlights his or her unusual, typically extraordinary, achievements that separate that person from the pack. This strategy is always beneficial.

3

Notice that I used the terms *unique* and *standard* in reference to applications and not applicants. This is because all premed students have the potential of being unique if they aren't already. But for some reason, many premeds mask their individuality and water down their rich experiences into a standard application, usually because they're afraid that they'll be identified as too unusual or strange for medical school. Unfortunately, they're wrong. Individuality is a highly valued commodity in the medical school admissions process. And this book will not only help you develop your own unique individuality but also, more important, help you present your unique individuality in an effective, noticeable application.

Compete on Your Own Terms

Don't merely try to compete with other applicants on their terms. Instead, find your own. By this, I mean, don't volunteer in a hospital simply because it's the recommended thing to do. There will always be someone else who's done it better and more often than you. Instead, spend your time pursuing your own personal, fulfilling goals. Travel abroad, study pottery, build a boat, learn about fishes or birds, take up photography, climb rocks at a local park, develop your racquetball game. Anything, as long as it's what you personally find enjoyable and you can stick with it long enough to gain some sort of recognition at it. By doing this, you're building up your own unique individuality and separating yourself from the pack.

Get Recognized

You're probably thinking that not everyone can be Volunteer of the Year or a champion tennis player or a concert pianist. But alas, my contention is that everyone can achieve some sort of distinction with a hobby. For example, instead of simply spending time swimming, work as a lifeguard or teach swimming classes at the YMCA. Instead of simply playing with clay, submit a few sculptures to local art shows. There are so many organizations and societies that sponsor so many events, it's hard not to find an outlet for your interests that won't eventually lead to some sort of productive display.

Keep this in mind: everyone who applies to medical school plays a decent game of tennis and can play a few tunes on the piano. But not everyone is a tennis instructor with a local youth group or an honorable mention pianist in the annual county recital. Find your niche and do it well. Otherwise, your list of hobbies on your application will look just like everyone else's.

Self-Diagnosis Exercise

Part A of this exercise lists some standard categories of information for medical school applicants. Fill in the blanks with what you think the standard premed applicant will have on his or her application. Space is provided in Part B for you to list information about yourself and your own accomplishments. On the lines in Part C, list the information and accomplishments from Part B that you believe would set your application apart from the usual premed application. In Part D, rank order the list you made in Part C to determine your unique individuality.

Part A: Standard Applicant Information and Accomplishments

Major _____

GPA _____

MCAT score _____

Academic honors and awards _____

Other awards _____

Volunteer work _____

Work experience _____

Club/organization membership _____

Hobbies/interests _____

Part B: My Application Information and Accomplishments

Major _____

GPA _____

MCAT score _____

Academic honors and awards _____

Other awards _____

Volunteer work _____

Work experience _____

Club/organization membership _____

Hobbies/interests _____

Part C: What Sets My Application Apart

_____

_____

_____

_____

_____

_____

Part D: My Unique Individuality

_____

_____

_____

_____

_____

_____

2 Do You Hate Biology?

Which major is best for you? If you're like most people, even most premed students, you might think that majoring in a hard life science (biology, chemistry, biochemistry) is a requirement of successful medical school admissions. This is absolutely wrong!

You can major in any subject you please. That's right, you can major in English, history, classics, romance languages, mathematics, computer science, sociology, American studies, anthropology, or anything else and still get into medical school. In fact, you may have a better chance of getting into medical school.

The general requirements for medical school are the following:

- One year of biological sciences
- One year of general chemistry
- One year of organic chemistry
- One year of physics
- One year of English

Some schools may require calculus or biochemistry, but those are exceptions. The above general requirements can easily be met with a minor or simple emphasis in science tacked on to a major in any field.

It's rumored that the physician-poet William Carlos Williams once said, "Those who major in science should be discouraged, even prohibited from pursuing medicine."

7

Egregious Error: When a student of mine discovered that I majored in philosophy in college, she said, "I wanted to major in French." She was, of course, a biology major. I asked her why she didn't, and she replied with the usual responses, "It's too late" (she was a college senior at the time), and "I didn't know I could." After a lengthy discussion of the pros and cons of switching her major this late in her studies, I offered her an automatic A in my course if she switched her major. Unfortunately, the prospect of spending one more semester making up her French major requirements didn't appeal to her; she didn't want to waste any more time before medical school than she had to. Imagine the lost opportunity—she could have been fluent in a second language, maybe spent some time overseas. But instead, she'll have to put off her interests for the rest of her life pursuing another goal in a completely unsatisfying and unnecessarily restrictive way.

I don't know who to blame when I run into the many students who tell me that they didn't know they could major in something other than a hard science. Should I blame them for not asking? Or should I blame the few people who actually tell unsuspecting students that they must carry a science major?

A 1992 study showed that students with "broad" backgrounds had no difference in overall scores on the national board exams, difficulty in medical school, specialty choice, or research careers when compared with "science" students (Koenig, 1992). Thus, a well-rounded, nonscience background will not adversely affect your medical school performance. In fact, it will increase your chances of admission.

Data from the Association of American Medical Colleges, presented in Table 2.1, show the undergraduate majors of the U.S. class entering in 1996. The table speaks for itself.

Think of it this way: Imagine you're an admissions dean at a medical school. Before you sit 5,000 applications. Biology, chemistry, or biochemistry majors make up 4,950 of the applications. The other 50 are scattered non-life-science majors. Which applications do you think will remain prominent in your mind and catch your attention? Your goal as a prospective student is to get your application noticed by the admissions committee. Carrying an unusual major may do the trick. So go ahead and major in French. Besides, you'll also enjoy your college time much more.

Table 2.1 clearly shows that students who carried nonscience majors performed as well, if not better, than their science colleagues. Some may take it

Table 2.1 Admissions Rates, by Selected Undergraduate Majors

Selected Undergrad Majors	Total Applicants	Accepted Applicants	
		Number	Percentage
Sciences			
Biology	17,713	6,163	35
Microbiology	1,092	357	33
Zoology	1,073	349	33
Biochemistry	2,732	1,160	43
Engineering[a]	1,559	661	42
Chemistry	2,709	1,049	39
Physics	300	127	42
Psychology	2,507	856	34
Nonsciences			
English	734	337	46
History	597	295	49
Philosophy	228	114	50
Other health professions			
Medical technology	276	56	20
Nursing	316	53	17
Pharmacy	317	83	26
Mixed disciplines			
Science double major	824	311	38
Nonscience double major	1,188	504	42
Interdisciplinary studies	253	137	54
1996 Total	46,968	17,385	37

SOURCE: Reprinted with permission from *Medical School Admissions Requirements, 1998-1999, United States and Canada,* published by the Association of American Medical Colleges.
a. Engineering category includes biomedical, chemical, and electrical.

too far and double-major in the sciences. Premeds are all overachievers, and they all subscribe to the "more is better" or "quantity > quality" theory of educational achievement. Personally, I think that a double major simply restricts one's academic choices even further by taking what should be a "minor" and elevating it to "major" status and thereby limiting the breadth of the transcript.

The point here is that majoring in a nonscience major such as urban planning and minoring in biology doesn't mean that you should pack your transcript with all UP and bio courses. Rather, take the required courses for your major, take the required premed courses for admissions, then spread out the rest of your time among all the other possibilities.

All students, regardless of major, should go through the college catalog and choose any course outside of their major that interests them and then do their best to take those courses in favor of other electives in their major. Don't be surprised if you become widely read, begin to develop interests in humanitarian causes, and start to have interesting conversations with everyone.

And besides, the above data show that science double majors have less chance of admission than nonscience single majors (38% vs. 48%).

As a final note on this subject, I am not at all encouraging those who truly enjoy the study of hard science to forego their interests and study the humanities simply for a statistical advantage in medical school admissions. By all means, if you love biology, major in it. But if you ever think that you might enjoy literature or music more, don't let the fear of medical school rejection stop you from changing your major.

Reference

Koenig, J. A. (1992). Comparison of medical school performances and career plans of students with broad and with science-focused premedical preparation. *Academic Medicine, 67,* 191-196.

3 Candy Striper?

It's common practice to seek volunteer time to "experience" the medical profession. So, in droves, premed students assault the volunteer offices of local hospitals hoping to obtain a peek at what it means to be a doctor. Most of these students wind up transporting patients from one ward to another, retrieving X rays from the radiology department, or observing a surgery from afar. There is usually a very weak correlation between volunteer work and doctor's work.

Egregious Error: Another student, a biology major with an average grade point average, worked in a lab one summer (sound familiar?) and came to me looking for advice. That summer, he planned on volunteering at a local, but nationally prominent, hospital. Why, I asked? Because, he revealed honestly, he thought it would help him get into medical school. Despite my advice, he went ahead and spent every Tuesday and Saturday at the hospital in the pediatric oncology ward. What was his volunteer assignment? He had to keep the playroom organized and clean and play with the kids when they came to visit the room. Kids, he figured, would be fun to play with. But of course, many of the kids were deathly ill and already had overprotective parents to play with.

At the end of the summer, after weeks of volunteering in the playroom, he confided that he had never met a physician or seen a patient from a physician's viewpoint, nor had he ever acquainted himself with any one patient long enough to understand his or her disease or situation. What did this experience tell him about the medical profession? All he could say was that he dreaded hospitals and sick people and that he had no idea what doctors did there. Was this a valuable experience?

If experience in the medical profession is really what you're looking for, you should find a practicing physician and follow him or her around in the office. Most will be too busy for you, but you may find one who's accommodating enough so that you learn what it really means to be a doctor, instead of learning what it means to merely take daily care of patient needs in the hospital, which is usually what volunteering in a hospital typically reveals. If you're insistent on volunteering in a hospital, make sure that you'll be working with physicians in a clinical setting—ideally, obtaining some hands-on patient care experience. Always ask yourself, "Am I learning something useful here, or am I a candy striper?"

Again, I'd like to emphasize that if you really get a kick out of volunteering your time in a hospital, go ahead and do it. But as with everything else, do it consistently and do it well. I knew one student who racked up 500 hours over the years at a local hospital and received its Volunteer of the Year award. She didn't mind transporting patients and cleaning bedpans because she did it for her own gratification, not simply to get into medical school. Needless to say, no one questioned her humanitarian concerns and she easily got accepted to medical school. Now, if you're thinking of volunteering one summer simply to round out your application for medical school, how will your few hours compare with this student's Volunteer of the Year award?

4 Researcher or Rat Killer?

Common practice also leads premed students to the nearest science lab to play with mice and other scientific equipment. Again, this chapter will explain all the pitfalls associated with wasting precious time as a "science slave" and will provide even more productive options.

Egregious Error: One student wanted to go to medical school, so he majored in biology, volunteered in a hospital, and decided to spend a summer working in a lab to "enhance his application," he told me. Did he want to pursue a career in medical or scientific research? Of course not. He wanted to be a practicing doctor; lab work was important, he acknowledged, but not for him. Yet he decided to spend an entire summer working in a lab.

What did he do? On Mondays, he killed mice and removed their pituitaries for one scientist, and from Tuesday to Friday, he removed eyeball lenses from chick embryos for another scientist. What did he get at the end of the summer? A few paychecks from a prominent laboratory, but that's it. He authored no publications, met no physicians (all the scientists in his lab had Ph.D.s), and thus received almost nothing to help him get into medical school.

When he asked for a recommendation letter from the lab chief, the letter basically said that the student "worked hard and performed his tasks well." Not exactly the glowing accolades that jump out to an admissions committee. How would a letter from his boss have differed if he'd spent the summer as employee of the month making deliveries for a local pizzeria?

The student almost mentioned that he received valuable work experience, but when asked, he had no idea what the lab did with those mouse pituitaries or with the chicken lenses for that matter. Finally, he admitted that outside of the money, he could've spent his summer doing something more productive or at least more fun.

Again, I want to emphasize that if you really love bench science, by all means, pursue your interests with a job in a laboratory. However, you must try to really make your experience count. By this, I mean that you should work in a lab that has a defined project well underway; get a job where you will be recognized as a contributor to that lab's work. Try as hard as you can to get into a project that will get you a published paper. By being published, you are showing the admissions committee that you actively participated in that lab's research and contributed your talents to their work. Otherwise, there's no way to tell if you were simply a beaker buffer or rat killer.

And be prepared to spend more than a few months with your research. Like all successful projects, results can't be expected after a few hours of work in one summer. Dedication and perseverance all pay off, so if you enjoy lab work, go for it consistently, either every summer or even on a regular part-time basis during classwork. If you really enjoy the work, it won't be difficult, and you'll definitely get some form of recognition in the end. Otherwise, you're just wasting your time.

5 More Is Better, Right?

Many applicants not only major in a science but often feel that more science classes on their transcript will boost their science grade point average (GPA) and also strike a chord in the heart of admissions committees. But I would like to make an appeal to the well-rounded, and even more important, well-educated student.

Egregious Error: One student majored in microbiology, volunteered in a hospital, and worked in a lab (does this sound redundant?). One summer, he decided that he would take two upper-level science courses to boost his science GPA (which was a respectable 3.5 out of 4.0 at the time) and thus make his transcript more competitive. I sat him in my office and placed a summer course catalog in front of him. I asked him to imagine that he was not applying to medical school or that he had already been accepted and to circle all the courses that he would like to take. Of course, he identified mostly history courses and other nonscience courses. I asked him why he didn't take these courses, and he frankly pointed out, "I need a higher GPA to get into medical school."

This student did win a volunteer award, so I encouraged him to keep going with his hospital work. But he wouldn't give up his holy grail of a significantly higher science GPA, even though we calculated that he would need three As in four-credit lab courses to improve his GPA by 0.1 point.

> This student ultimately did not change his major, even though he admitted to a passion for history. Coincidentally, he went through four years of college and didn't take a single history course. Who knows what would've happened to him if he'd taken a few history courses and pursued his interest in medieval political theory instead of spending a summer memorizing facts about amoeba?

A perpetual assumption among most premed students is that a higher science GPA is always desirable. But I have to ask, at what price? College is typically only four years long, and the explicit requirements for medical school admissions consist of a select, but small, number of basic science courses. What's the solution? Obviously, you need to shoot for the best grades your first time around in the basic courses. The key here is quality, not quantity. If you succeed at the basic courses, you won't have to rely on the "extra science crutch" that many students wrongly take for granted.

For students interested in beefing up their science GPA, I typically ask them to calculate how much their GPA will increase with As in a few extra science courses. Usually, the answer is "not very much." Or I ask them what their reasonably ideal GPA would be and how many As they'd require to achieve that number. Usually the answer to this question is, "Yikes!"

• **Should I ever take more science?** There is only one instance when extra science courses will be of any benefit to a student. If your performance in the basic required courses is poor, you can prove your academic mettle to the admissions committee by taking upper-level science courses and getting As in them. But you run the risk of getting identical or even worse grades in these presumably tougher courses. And I've seen many students run into this trap. Very few students are successful at this strategy. Also, there's enough room within the basic courses themselves to prove your mettle. If you got a B in general chemistry, an A in organic chemistry will surely settle any questions of your chemistry aptitude. A grade of C in freshman biology followed by an A in junior physics may indicate continued maturity. No need to stock up on more advanced biology courses to directly "make up" for a poor showing on your first try.

• **Don't repeat courses.** The worst thing to do would be to repeat the same basic courses in an attempt to get a higher grade. Most schools won't replace your previous grade with your new one, and generous schools will simply average the two. In fact, the American Medical College Application Service (AMCAS—more on this later) requires that you list both grades and average the two in your GPA calculation. Again, the perilous risk of identical or worse grades exists.

If you're diligent enough to get As in all the basic required courses, extra science courses are no more helpful, perhaps even more harmful, than a transcript sporting a variety of coursework from disparate departments. I encourage history, philosophy, education, sociology, economics, even physical education for all students. Some may think that taking advanced courses will help them get ahead in medical school, but they're seriously mistaken: If advanced courses will assist in medical school, then medical schools would accept advanced standing for the more "accomplished" students, yet none do so. In addition, they're seriously ignoring the point of an undergraduate education, which is not simply to get ahead in medical school but, rather, to broaden your mind and develop your sense of humanity.

• **Health backgrounds aren't everything.** Don't be fooled into thinking that students who have health-related activities on their application have a better chance at admissions than those who do not. There is no reason for a medical school to accept someone with numerous health-related courses or hobbies over someone with identical achievements in non-health-related fields. This is especially true if the student with a bevy of health-related experience has no evidence of distinction in them. Why would a medical school accept a plain old hospital-volunteering, lab-working science student instead of an award-winning community theater actor with a major in Spanish? If they've both completed the required science prerequisites, well, then the atypical candidate is more likely to get noticed by the admissions committee. Think about it.

• **Aren't grades enough?** Absolutely not. The admissions director at a prestigious medical school told me that he could fill his entire freshman class with 4.0s in biomedical engineering—or entirely with Ph.D.s, for that matter. That, in fact, is what makes the admissions decisions so difficult. Schools are trying to find a diverse body of students who represent various backgrounds and experiences. Excellent grades are by no means your sole ticket to admissions.

The main point of Chapters 2, 3, and 4 is this: Don't waste your time doing something you don't like simply for the sake of getting into medical school.

If you don't like what you're doing, it'll eventually show, either through poor performance, frustration, or worst of all, lost time that you could've spent doing something you really enjoy. On the other hand, if you truly pursue your interests with gusto and energy, you will eventually reap the rewards of a fun job well done. And you'll probably be a better person, too. Or as many applicants remind me, you'll be a better person who also has a better chance of being admitted to medical school.

6 Older and Wiser

This chapter is dedicated to the postbaccalaureate applicant who has been out of school for many years, perhaps in another career. These unique applicants need unique advice.

The first question that postbaccalaureate students ask is, "What're my chances?" My reply is always, "Excellent!" I say this because the postbaccalaureate student typifies an application with unique individuality. Most have already embarked on successful careers, started families, and raised children. By virtue of life experience alone, they are already a breed apart.

Many medical schools admit several older, second-career students (Case Western Reserve University calls them "bent arrows") because they definitely supply a dose of variety to the student body. But there's never a quota or special admissions program for postbaccalaureate students; they're admitted simply because they exhibit strong unique individuality characteristics that distinguish themselves from the other standard applicants.

The **general principle** for postbaccalaureate applicants is the same as for typical applicants: Identify your unique individuality and amplify it in your application. Most postbaccalaureates applicants are lucky in that they have a plethora of life experiences on which to base their unique individuality. The one trick they have to master is explaining why they now want to pursue medicine as a career.

For example, if you're a postbaccalaureate and you've just spent five years as a manager in a successful auto parts company, you'll be hard-pressed to convince an admissions dean that you've always wanted to be a doctor. The question you'll want to answer is, "Why would you want to give up a successful career for perhaps a more tenuous one?" Another of the admissions committee's main questions will be, "Why did you wait?"

Also, if you've been unsuccessful at a particular career, admissions deans will not want to hear that "I couldn't make it as a cosmetics salesperson, so I'll do something easier like medicine." Of course, that's exaggerating, but you'd be surprised how many subtle variations of that theme tend to wind up in more than a few postbaccalaureate applications.

Previous careers, regardless of their relationship or nonrelationship to medicine or science, should never be shamefully hidden or obscured. Instead, they should be used as a way to color your experience and add to your sense of unique individuality. The key is to explain your interest in transitioning from them to medicine. In general, postbaccalaureates applicants must come up with solid reasons for why they want to enter the medical profession and why they want to enter it now.

How should a postbaccalaureate applicant without a science background go about fulfilling the prerequisites? There are two options: Take the individual courses piecemeal at your local college or university, or enroll in a formal postbaccalaureate program. There are no data to indicate that one path finds more success than another. Usually, the decision comes down to convenience, tuition, advice, and location.

Formal Postbaccalaureate Programs

Some colleges and universities offer formalized courses of study for students who have already completed a bachelor's degree (or more) in a nonscience field or who are returning for refresher science courses after numerous years away from the field. Bear in mind the following points when considering a formal program.

• **Academic advantage?** Formal postbaccalaureate premed programs provide no academic advantage to simply taking piecemeal coursework at your local state university. Ask yourself, if one school offers the same course within a formal postbaccalaureate program as well as a part-time, nondegree option, what's the difference? Usually there is none. Your transcript will reflect the exact same course.

• **Advising advantage?** Formal postbaccalaureate programs usually do provide an adviser or group of advisers who have experience with postbaccalaureate applicants. These advisers will personally become familiar with you, your academic history, and your application. If your adviser knows what he or she is doing, this alone will provide you with an advantage by establishing a relationship with one person so that your talents and qualities will be well promoted in your application.

But keep in mind that most college and universities have premedical advisers available to you, regardless of your enrollment status. Thus, simply being a part-time nondegree student still allows you to take advantage of any premedical advisers who may be available. Again, there's no guarantee that one method provides any obvious advantages.

• **Financial folly?** Typically, the most important factor in making the postbaccalaureate decision is the cost of tuition. If you are considering a formal program, you must carefully research their costs. Do yourself a favor and compare it with the cost of obtaining identical coursework at a local state university. Chances are, your costs will be much cheaper outside the formal program. Education is a pricey commodity these days; you wouldn't drive a car off the lot before shopping around, so do your homework before you plunk down a hefty deposit on your medical career. The third book in this series, *The Right Price* by Christine Wiebe, offers good advice on the financial considerations of going to medical school.

• **Guaranteed?** Many formal postbaccalaureate programs advertise themselves as having a particular success rate. How is this possible? Some of the more successful programs weed out "unfavorable" candidates by accepting only those students who already have successful academic credentials. Some programs designed to award master's degrees even offer "guaranteed" enrollment in a medical school if high grades are attained in certain classes. There's no such thing. Don't be duped.

• **Social advantages?** One advantage to a formal postbaccalaureate program may be the company of other postbaccalaureate students. When you're in the trenches, it's always reassuring to have fellow premeds for commiseration. These benefits are immeasurable, but again, you must decide if this is something you value. But many larger universities also have large numbers of postbaccalaureate students, some of whom have begun social organizations. Chances are, if you look around, you'll be surprised at what you might find.

• **Schedule advantages?** Some programs provide coursework within a compacted time frame and go out of their way to accommodate the admissions cycle as best they can. But their ability to accommodate your schedule is limited by their enrollment numbers and every other student's schedule. Again, you should compare any formal program's schedule with one at your local university. Either way, you'll find just as much flexibility to fit your needs.

Ultimately, the decision to enroll in a formal program, as opposed to taking individual courses yourself, is your own. I urge you to gather information and investigate the possibilities as well as the costs and requirements before making your final decision.

There are so many formal programs for postbaccalaureate students (at least 100), it would be impractical to list them here. However, a comprehensive, up-to-date list can be found on the Internet at the Association of American Medical Colleges Website: http://www.aamc.org/stuapps/appinfo/post-bac.htm

Some programs specifically seek out underrepresented minority students, economically disadvantaged students, state residents, or those who have already applied unsuccessfully to medical school. All the peculiarities of each program are mentioned at this site. Definitely worth visiting.

Quit Your Hurrying!

With regards to your applications and schedule, again, it's up to you how you want to proceed. All the other advice in this book can be applied to you as well—for example, take an early MCAT (Chapter 7), eschew Early D (Chapter 16), carefully research your schools, and so on.

Egregious Error: One postbaccalaureate student had no science background and decided to take the basic science courses at the local college. However, she decided to take them all at once. Imagine, General Chemistry I, Organic Chemistry I, Principles of Physics I, all in one semester!

She also admitted that she'd not only disliked the sciences as an undergraduate but that she'd tried a few courses back then and performed poorly. As expected, she performed poorly this time, too. The course difficulty was tripled by taking them all at the same time.

One problem that many postbaccalaureates applicants encounter is a sense of urgency. Not only do they want to jettison their current career, they want to replace it with a medical career as soon as possible. Don't fall into this trap. You must remain levelheaded and reasonable. If you have no science background whatsoever, you should expect about two full calendar years of preparation, examination, and application before beginning medical school. If you have some science background, you may be able to shorten that time.

Don't try to cram courses into shortened schedules by carrying an unreasonable course load or by taking advanced classes without prerequisites. Rushing through important prerequisite courses typically results in errors at your expense. The best thing to do is to create a calendar and schedule with reasonable goals, then stick to it. As stated in the first section of this book, preparation is everything.

Section II
In the Thick of It

Now that we've covered the ground with regard to your premedical preparation, this section will detail all the steps in the actual medical school application process and provide advice on avoiding the common mistakes. Remember that every single step in the medical school application procedures is an opportunity for horrific mistakes. Don't trip up!

7 The MCAT

The MCAT is the dreaded exam, probably the most stressful exam for all physicians, because this exam actually may determine whether or not you get into medical school. The subsequent exams (boards, specialty exams) pale in comparison with the stress and anxiety caused by this baby.

• **MCAT registration.** You can get registration forms for the Medical College Admissions Test from your college premedical adviser or from the MCAT offices at this address:

Medical College Admissions Test
P.O. Box 4056
Iowa City, IA 52243
(319) 337-1357

• **When should I take the MCAT?** The MCAT is offered twice a year, in April and in August. When you should take the test depends on when you want to begin medical school. Typically, the premed student takes the MCAT in the spring of the junior year of college after completing the bulk of basic premed courses, applies in the summer between junior and senior years, gets accepted in the winter/spring of senior year, and relaxes until medical school starts next fall. Thus, the MCAT is taken a full one and a half calendar years before you begin medical school, and at the very least before you apply to medical school.

• **Spring or fall?** All premeds should take the spring MCAT in preparation for a summer application. Premeds should take the fall MCAT *only* if they're planning on applying the summer afterward. If you take the fall MCAT, your applications will be placed on hold until your scores are reported, sometime in October. There's no point in applying early if your applications simply sit in a pile for months awaiting your MCAT score. Also, your scores may affect which medical schools you apply to. If you apply to several highly competitive schools and fare poorly on your fall MCATs, not only is your application already late, but it's not competitive. That's two strikes against you. Conversely, if you score higher than expected, you are behind in applying to more competitive schools, where abundant early and competitive applications are the norm. And having your applications in place before your exam will place additional burdens on your test-taking skills. If you want every advantage in your favor, you need to have all your ducks in a row before you apply.

• **Can I apply before the fall MCAT?** Medical schools typically do not require MCAT scores before you can submit an application. However, they do require your MCAT scores before they can offer you an acceptance. You can officially submit your application without MCAT scores anytime before the fall test date, but your admissions decision will be delayed until your MCAT scores arrive around October. As explained above, applying before your MCAT scores arrive leaves all your efforts in limbo. Should you defer applying an entire year so that you can take the spring MCAT before submitting an application? That decision is up to you and is determined by the overall quality of your application. Don't hurry. Plan ahead. Take the MCAT at least in the spring before you apply.

• **MCAT before coursework?** Some premeds take the MCAT before they've completed their basic premedical coursework. Although admissions committees may take a low MCAT score into consideration if the coursework hasn't been completed yet, this is not the kind of attention you want to bring to yourself during the admissions process. You should complete at least the bulk of your premedical coursework before taking the exam.

• **MCAT review courses.** There are several commercial review courses for the MCAT, as well as local courses available at individual colleges and universities. The decision to enroll in one of these courses is a difficult one, but it is usually determined by answering two simple questions: "Do I need more structure in my studying pattern?" "Can I afford this course?"

There are plenty of "practice MCAT" books and thousands of practice questions available in your local bookstore. But many students wind up with several unopened books sitting on their desk until a few nights before the exam. A review course may help you in keeping to a strict schedule, preventing "cramming" when it's already too late.

Review courses cost a pretty penny. On one hand, you may not want to take chances with the most important exam in your life. Many students wish they'd forked out the cash after they receive poor scores. On the other hand, if you're a good student and have developed good study skills, a prep course may not provide you with much of an advantage. Some students wonder if they could've saved the dough after receiving good scores. You know your own financial situation better than anyone, so the decision is entirely up to you. Based on the significant cost of such courses, this is not a decision to be made lightly.

For those who decide not to enroll in a review course, there are ways to obtain the same benefits on your own. You can plan a study course with a group of fellow premeds and thus keep each other on an adequate study schedule. You can also obtain any of the available practice MCAT test books and take the tests in groups, timing yourself for practice.

• **Should I release my scores?** When you take the MCAT, you will have the opportunity to release your scores to all schools. There is *no reason* for you not to release your scores to the medical schools. If you do not release your scores, schools will still know that you've taken the MCAT but decided not to release your scores. Again, this is not the kind of attention you want to bring to yourself. If you score poorly, there is no benefit in hiding your scores; you will absolutely not receive any sort of admission without them. And if you score very poorly, schools will see your improvement when you release your next score results because all previous scores are reported with the most recent ones. If you score well, you won't need to take the MCAT again, so these are the scores you'll have to release. Release them. End of story.

• **No MCAT necessary?** Some unusual medical schools (notably Johns Hopkins) do not require an MCAT test score at all. However, they do require some form of standardized test score such as the SAT (Scholastic Aptitude Test), ACT (America College Test), GRE (Graduate Record Exam), or even an MCAT score if you're so inclined. This requirement exists because there are many standardized tests that lie ahead on the road to being a physician. Not gauging your ability in standardized tests ignores a major qualification

Table 7.1   Average 1997 MCAT Scores

Subject	All 1997 Test Takers	1997 Accepted Test Takers
Biological science	9	10
Physical science	9	10
Verbal reasoning	9	10
Writing sample	O	P
Average total	27	30

SOURCE: Association of American Medical Colleges Web page:
http://www.aamc.org/stuapps/admiss/mcat/mcat9297.htm

for success as a physician. For practical purposes, you should never bank on getting in to a medical school that doesn't require the MCATs. The odds are simply too great against you. You will have to take the MCAT.

• **Med-MAR.** The Medical Minority Applicant Registry (Med-MAR) is a program that provides information on minority applicants to medical schools. Underrepresented students may register for Med-MAR when they take the MCAT. Med-MAR simply provides information on registered students to medical schools who are interested in creating a diverse student body. Most medical schools actively attempt to create a diverse student body, especially in compliance with the AAMC's (Association of American Medical Colleges)"3000 by 2000" initiative. By all means, if you qualify for Med-MAR, register. Consider it a recruitment tool free of charge.

• **Should I try again?** A good MCAT score is great, but what happens if the score is mediocre or even below average? Table 7.1 shows the average scores (and standard deviations) in 1997 for all MCAT takers. As expected, those students who ultimately received an acceptance and enrolled had a higher MCAT score on average than the total group. These data also indicate that 9s and 10s should be your goal on each section of the MCAT.

The scores you need are those that correlate with your GPA. In other words, if you have an average science GPA (around 3.5 for successful applicants), then your MCAT scores should hover around 10s. If you have a higher GPA, your MCAT score should be accordingly higher. A low MCAT score with a high GPA will be interpreted poorly, and this is a situation you must avoid. Likewise, if you have a lower GPA, your MCAT score is expected to be lower. **This is your opportunity.** With a lower GPA, a higher-than-average MCAT score may indicate inherent ability under stress. However, you must never assume that a high MCAT score makes up for or legitimizes a low GPA. There is never such a guarantee.

If you have lower than expected MCAT scores, you may take the MCAT again, but remember that you do so at the risk of scoring even lower on the next exam. Keep in mind that all previous MCAT scores are always reported with your most recent scores, so there's no way to hide any scores from medical schools. Low, or even average MCAT scores, followed by even lower scores are disastrous for your application. If you do decide to retake the MCAT, you must plan a serious course of study to improve your score.

One interesting study (Koenig & Leger, 1997) seemed to indicate that students who used a commercial review course were more likely to have improved retest scores. But again, there's no way to tell if prep courses are merely markers for those who are already well motivated and financially well-off. But remember, the best way to prevent taking the MCAT a second time is to prepare seriously and well for the first time. Don't slack off.

• **Special permission after three.** You must apply for special permission to take the MCAT if you have taken the test three or more times since 1977. To receive permission, you need to prove that you're actively applying to a medical school, either with a completed application, letter of rejection, or letter from a medical school or adviser. This documentation is required each time you want to retake the test. Requests will be reviewed and permission confirmed in writing prior to the test date. For more information, contact the MCAT Program Office at the address given earlier in this chapter.

Reference

Koenig, J. A., & Leger, K. F. (1997). A comparison of retest performance and rest-preparation methods for MCAT examinees grouped by gender and race-ethnicity. *Academic Medicine, 25,* 2-4.

8 M.D. or D.O.?

Many of you may have no idea what an osteopathic physician is, but this chapter will try to dispel myths and answer some questions about D.O.s and their important role in modern medical practice.

What Is an Osteopathic Physician?

The most obvious difference between osteopathic and allopathic physicians is the letters after their name. Osteopathic physicians have a Doctor of Osteopathy (D.O.) degree instead of a Medical Doctor (M.D.) degree. But following is a comparison of their similarities and differences, theoretical and practical.

• **Similarities.** The modern osteopathic medical school curriculum is quite similar to the allopathic curriculum. Osteopathic students have to pass anatomy, physiology, pathology, and all the clinical clerkships identical to allopathic students. As a fond saying goes, osteopathic physicians use the same books, see the same diseases in the same patients, compete for the same residencies, get the same license, dispense the same medicines, and get paid the same money. The federal government (i.e., the people who reimburse doctors for Medicare) and the American Medical Association both recognize no difference between D.O.s and M.D.s. Osteopaths practice in every specialty from neurosurgery to family practice, in settings from hospitals to clinics, and are eligible for full medical and surgical licenses in all 50 states. In fact, the state of California offered D.O.s an M.D. degree for a small fee during the 1950s. That alone should say enough about their similarities.

• **Differences.** Osteopathic medicine began formally in 1892 by Andrew Still, M.D., a physician who wanted to create a more comprehensive, holistic approach to medicine based on the belief that the human body is capable of healing itself and that there is a musculoskeletal component to every disease. This philosophy continues today in the osteopathic curriculum where, in addition to the standard medical coursework, students are taught osteopathic manipulative technique (OMT). Osteopathic physicians focus on the musculoskeletal system, as it reflects and influences the condition of the entire body. Thus, OMT is used to diagnose as well as to treat certain conditions, either on its own or in combination with other therapies, such as medicines or surgery.

Osteopathic physicians compose 10% of the physician population, serve 20% of our underserved communities, and have historically chosen primary care practice in large numbers.

For all intents and purposes, there is little difference between a D.O. and an M.D. Every premed student should consider osteopathic medical schools alongside allopathic medical schools when determining their schools of choice.

For more information about osteopathic medicine and osteopathic medical schools, you can contact the following organizations dedicated to osteopathic medicine.

American Association of Colleges of Osteopathic Medicine
5550 Friendship Boulevard, Suite 310
Chevy Chase, MD 20815-7231
Main: (301) 968-4100
http://www.aacom.org

Student Osteopathic Medical Association
142 East Ontario Street
Chicago, IL 60611
(800) 237-SOMA
http://www.studentdoctor.com/

American Osteopathic Association
142 E. Ontario Street
Chicago, IL 60611
(800) 621-1773
E-mail: osteomed@wwa.com
http://www.am-osteo-assn.org

9 They're All the Same, Aren't They?

Choosing a medical school is a difficult task. Sure, everyone knows that Johns Hopkins is a prestigious school and that your state school probably has the least expensive tuition for you. But not many people know enough about unique programs within each medical school that may significantly enhance your academic experience.

Yes, it is true that every medical school adheres to rigorous curriculum and accreditation standards such that all graduates are qualified to go on to residency and practice medicine. The old joke that 50% of America's doctors graduated in the bottom half of their class doesn't take into account that every medical school graduate is at least minimally competent in patient care, regardless of where he or she went to school.

But most people do react one way when you tell them you went to Harvard and differently when you tell them you went to the University of Massachusetts. Sure, that's a prestige question, but there are differences between medical schools that go beyond competitive admissions. Every medical school is good enough to train you to be a physician. In that sense, they are all identical. However, significant differences may exist between schools. These qualities should be explored and used **to your advantage** in the application process because they may play a role in your being accepted or rejected. This chapter will lay out some of these differences for you and show you how to use these differences to your advantage.

35

Egregious Error: One student came to me for advice after he submitted his applications. His first choice was Cornell. When I asked why, he replied confidently, "I applied to Cornell 'cos I love Ithaca, man; it's a beautiful town. Have you ever been there?"

I could only say, "No, but I've been to New York City. Why didn't you apply to any New York schools?"

"Too much crime, and it's dirty." I had to break it to him gently: "Well, New York City . . . that's where Cornell's medical school is." He appeared stunned as he realized that the undergraduate and medical school campuses of Cornell were in two different places.

Yes, the above is a true story. Imagine if he had applied to Cornell Early D (see chapter 16) and been accepted? Moral of the story? **Research your medical schools before you apply to them.** Sounds simple, but you'd be surprised.

Is Your Medical School Prepared for the 21st Century?

In 1910, Abraham Flexner, M.D., published an investigative report for the Carnegie Foundation evaluating medical education. He basically stated that most medical schools trained doctors poorly. This report prescribed the blueprint for today's curriculum—that is, two years of basic sciences and two years of clinical work in a hospital. The Flexner report became a benchmark in medical education history. Unfortunately, the same curriculum has remained mostly intact for the last 90 years. Although no formal Flexner report has been published recently, many medical schools have begun tampering with their curriculum in the last 15 or so years. Consider this an implicit acknowledgment that medical education in the United States needs to change to produce better physicians for the modern health care system.

You've probably heard of problem-based learning and primary care, two catchphrases in medical education nowadays. Most every medical school is tampering somewhat with their curriculum, and some are offering truly innovative and unique programs for their students. Here are some of the more common trends touted by individual medical schools as "innovations." Don't be swayed easily by any such advertisement into thinking that a particular program is unique because of these now-dated features. The approaches to medical education listed below have become fairly standard; the archaic medical school without any such innovations is an anachronism awaiting disaccreditation.

• **Early patient contact.** It only makes sense that a medical school should require experience in patient care early in the first year. Why should students wait until biochemistry is mastered before they can practice talking to people?

Most medical schools are touting patient contact early in their curricula, ranging from simple history-taking experiences to "shadowing" a physician longitudinally. The most optimal opportunity is a longitudinal experience with one physician so that you can follow patients over an extended period of time, thereby observing the course of their disease. By 1999, if a medical school does not require patient contact beginning in the first year, they're way behind.

If you consider yourself a "people person" who thrives on person-to-person interactions, a curriculum with early extended patient contact may provide you with an opportunity to show your colors.

• **Problem-based learning.** Like most catchphrases, problem-based learning (PBL, also known as case-based or self-directed learning) means different things to different people, especially in medical school. The general definition is the presentation of a patient case or problem that requires students to pursue the answer through independent study, collaborative education, and book research.

Almost every medical school has some form of PBL, usually as a part of its overall curriculum. If a school does not have any sort of PBL as a requirement for its students, the students are probably still sitting in a lecture hall built in 1910, napping soundly.

If you have an affinity for independent study and teaching others what you've learned, extensive PBL curricula may be your forte.

• **Primary care.** Primary care is another catchphrase that means different things to different people. Some schools consider an outpatient clinic in a tertiary care hospital to be a primary care experience; others define primary care experience as an inpatient rotation in a community hospital.

Entire books have attempted to define primary care, but for the purposes of this guide, let primary care be defined as a *required* outpatient family practice rotation. And to be effective, the family medicine rotation should be completed in the third year—typically, before the student has firmly decided on a career specialty choice.

Some schools may require a primary care elective in the fourth year, revealing plenty about the school, because most students have made their career choices by the end of third year. Would you attend a law school that didn't require a course in contracts before the last semester? Medical schools that do not require a family medicine rotation in the third year are significantly limiting the educational opportunities for their students.

If primary care is your desired career track, you should pursue schools that promote significant primary care experiences throughout their curriculum. And if you want a balanced education that offers you a sampling of every major specialty, a required third-year family medicine rotation should be on your list of must-haves.

• **Computer-based learning.** Computers allow physicians and medical students to perform tasks that couldn't be done 10 years ago. Hence, Computer-Based Learning is another trend in modern medical education. Computers are replacing animal labs, preparing students for gross anatomy dissections, taking the place of standard written exams, and even simulating patient care scenarios. However, computers are costly, and not every medical school has the wherewithal to provide an adequate supply of computers and software for every student. Computers will be a significant part of medical practice in the 21st century, and medical schools should provide this basic competency for future physicians.

If you are already familiar with computers and computer applications, a curriculum with computer-based learning options may help you flourish. Also, if you've never touched a computer before, a hefty dose of computer-based learning is the best way to prepare you for the real world.

• **Systems-based learning.** In the old days, medical students would learn everything about one basic science (e.g., anatomy), then move on to another subject (e.g., physiology). A systems-based learning program teaches the complete functioning and pathology of one body system (e.g., gastrointestinal or musculoskeletal) and combines all the disparate traditional basic science disciplines into that module. It's one easy way of arranging scattered information into a sensible pattern.

Combined-Degree Programs

Modern medicine isn't just about taking care of individual patients. In fact, more students are interested in obtaining further training to enhance their medical education. What does this say about medical education?

There is no law that prohibits those with an M.D. degree from later enrolling in another graduate or professional school. However, many medical schools have combined-degree programs that may offer the benefits of reduced total required years of study for both degrees and/or reduced tuition for both degrees.

If you think you have interests that combine another profession with medicine, consider the following combined-degree programs.

• **M.D./D.O. with Ph.D, or M.A. or M.S.** Typically, these programs are designed for the academic physician who wants to pursue a research career. The additional degree requirements, which may take from three to five years, are usually carried out between the second and third year of the standard curriculum. The Ph.D. degrees are usually offered in standard basic science disciplines, such as anatomy, physiology, pathology, immunology, and so on. However, some programs offer master's degrees and degrees in other non-science subjects. In fact, the University of Chicago has a separate M.D.-Ph.D. track for those people wishing to pursue an advanced degree in the humanities as it relates to medicine. Contact each school (see Table 9.1) for more information about their specific degree opportunities and requirements.

• **Medical scientist training program.** The medical scientist training program (MSTP) is basically an M.D.-Ph.D. program supported financially by the National Institutes of Health. There are approximately 150 MSTP positions available each year at 33 participating medical schools. Competition is stiff, but those who are selected receive full tuition and a $10,000 per year stipend. Did you ever imagine you'd *make* money during medical school? The schools listed in Table 9.2 offer the MSTP program.

For more information on the MSTP, contact the individual schools listed in Table 9.2 or the National Institutes of Health Medical Scientist Training Program.

Table 9.1   Combined M.D.-Ph.D. and D.O.-Ph.D. Programs

Alabama
  University of Alabama School of Medicine
  University of South Alabama
Arizona
  University of Arizona
Arkansas
  University of Arkansas
California
  University of California, Davis
  University of California, Irvine
  University of California, Los Angeles
  University of California, San Diego
  University of California, San Francisco
  Loma Linda University
  University of Southern California
  Stanford University
Colorado
  University of Colorado
Connecticut
  University of Connecticut
  Yale University
Florida
  University of Florida
  University of Miami
Georgia
  Emory University
  Medical College of Georgia
  Morehouse School of Medicine
Hawaii
  University of Hawaii
Illinois
  Chicago Medical School
  University of Chicago
  University of Illinois, Chicago
  University of Illinois, Urbana-Champaign
  Loyola-Stritch School of Medicine
  Northwestern University
  Rush Medical College
Indiana
  University of Indiana
Iowa
  University of Iowa
Kansas
  University of Kansas
Kentucky
  University of Kentucky
  University of Louisville

Louisiana
  Louisiana State University—New Orleans
  Louisiana State University—Shreveport
  Tulane University
Maryland
  Johns Hopkins University
  University of Maryland
Massachusetts
  Boston University
  Harvard Medical School
  University of Massachusetts
  Tufts University
Michigan
  Michigan State University
  Michigan State Osteopathic
  University of Michigan
  Wayne State University
Minnesota
  Mayo Medical School
  University of Minnesota—Minneapolis
Mississippi
  University of Mississippi
Missouri
  University of Missouri—Columbia
  University of Missouri—Kansas City
  University of St. Louis
  Washington University (St. Louis)
Nebraska
  Creighton University
  University of Nebraska Medical Center
Nevada
  University of Nevada
New Hampshire
  Dartmouth Medical School
New Jersey
  UMDNJ—New Jersey Medical
  UMDNJ—Robert Wood Johnson
New York
  Albany Medical College
  Albert Einstein University
  Columbia University
  Cornell University Medical College
  Mount Sinai School of Medicine
  New York College of Osteopathic Medicine
  New York Medical College
  New York University
  University of Rochester

State University of New York (SUNY)—
  Brooklyn
State University of New York (SUNY)—
  Buffalo
State University of New York (SUNY)—
  Stony Brook
State University of New York (SUNY)—
  Syracuse
North Carolina
  Duke University
  East Carolina University
  University of North Carolina
North Dakota
  University of North Dakota
Ohio
  Case Western Reserve University
  University of Cincinnati
  Medical College of Ohio
  Ohio State University
  Ohio College of Osteopathic Medicine
  Wright State University
Oklahoma
  University of Oklahoma
Oregon
  University of Oregon
Pennsylvania
  Thomas Jefferson University
  Allegheny University of the Health
    Sciences
  Pennsylvania State University
  University of Pennsylvania
  University of Pittsburgh
  Temple University
Rhode Island
  Brown University
South Carolina
  Medical University of South Carolina
  University of South Carolina
South Dakota
  University of South Dakota

Tennessee
  Meharry Medical College
  University of Tennessee—Memphis
  Vanderbilt University
Texas
  Baylor University
  Texas A&M
  Texas College of Osteopathic Medicine
  Texas Tech
  University of Texas—Galveston
  University of Texas—Houston
  University of Texas—San Antonio
  University of Texas—Southwestern
Utah
  University of Utah
Vermont
  University of Vermont
Virginia
  Eastern Virginia Medical School
  Medical College of Virginia
  University of Virginia
Washington
  University of Washington—Seattle
Washington, D.C.
  George Washington University
  Georgetown University
  Howard University
West Virginia
  Marshall University
  West Virginia University
Wisconsin
  Medical College of Wisconsin
  University of Wisconsin
Canada
  Dalhousie University
  University of Toronto
  McGill University
  University of Montreal (M.D.-M.S.C. and
    M.D.-Ph.D.)
  University of Sherbrooke (M.D.-M.S.C.
    and M.D.-Ph.D.)

Table 9.2   Medical Scientist Training Programs

University of Alabama	University of Michigan
Albert Einstein College of Medicine (New York)	University of Minnesota
	Mount Sinai School of Medicine (New York)
Baylor College of Medicine	New York University
University of California—Los Angeles	State University of New York (SUNY)—
University of California—San Diego	Stony Brook
University of California—San Francisco	Northwestern University (Illinois)
Case Western Reserve University (Ohio)	University of Pennsylvania
University of Chicago	University of Pittsburgh
University of Colorado	University of Rochester (New York)
Columbia University (New York)	Stanford University (California)
Cornell University Medical School (New York)	University of Texas Southwestern
	Tufts University (Massachusetts)
Duke University (North Carolina)	Vanderbilt University (Tennessee)
Emory University (Georgia)	University of Virginia
Harvard Medical School (Massachusetts)	Washington University (St. Louis)
University of Iowa	University of Washington (Seattle)
Johns Hopkins University (Maryland)	Yale University (Connecticut)

National Institutes of Health
Medical Scientist Training Program
Room 905, Westwood Building
Bethesda, Maryland, 20892
(301) 594-7744

Table 9.3 lists several other schools with formal combined-degree programs. Of course, you can always create your own combined-degree program. Look around and seek out the possibilities; you never know what you'll find for yourself.

The most complete catalog of allopathic medical schools is the Association of American Medical College's (AAMC) *Curriculum Directory* and *Medical School Admissions Requirements.* The American Association of Colleges of Osteopathic Medicine (AACOM) publishes their *Annual Statistical Report* and their *College Information Booklet,* which describe each of the osteopathic medical schools and provide data on curricula, student characteristics, tuition and fees, and so on. You can find copies of these books at your premedical adviser's office or in your school library. Get them and give them a good read. What you'll find may surprise you.

Table 9.3   Other Combined-Degree Programs

M.D. or D.O. with M.B.A.
   Allegheny University of the Health Sciences (Pennsylvania)
   University of California, Davis
   University of California, Irvine
   University of California, Los Angeles
   Case Western Reserve University (Ohio)
   University of Chicago
   Dartmouth Medical School (New Hampshire)
   University of Illinois, Urbana-Champaign
   McGill University (Canada)
   New York College of Osteopathic Medicine
   Northwestern University (M.D.-M.M.) (Illinois)
   University of Pennsylvania
   Philadelphia College of Osteopathic Medicine (with St. Joseph's University)
   Thomas Jefferson Medical College (Pennsylvania)
   Tufts University (with Northeastern and Brandeis) (Massachusetts)
   Vanderbilt University (Tennessee)
   Wake Forest University School of Medicine (North Carolina)
M.D.-J.D. Programs
   Case Western Reserve University (Ohio)
   University of Chicago
   Duke University (North Carolina)
   University of Illinois, Urbana-Champaign
   University of Pennsylvania
   Southern Illinois University
   West Virginia University
   Yale University School of Medicine (Connecticut)
M.D. or D.O. with M.P.H.
   University of Arizona
   Boston University
   University of California, Davis
   University of California, San Francisco
   Columbia University (New York)
   Duke University (North Carolina)
   Emory University (Georgia)
   George Washington University (Washington, D.C.)
   University of Michigan
   Morehouse School of Medicine (Georgia)
   Mount Sinai (M.S. in Community Medicine) (New York)
   UMDNJ—Robert Wood Johnson (New Jersey)
   University of North Carolina—Chapel Hill
   Northwestern University (Illinois)
   Nova Southeastern Osteopathic Medicine (Florida)
   Philadelphia College of Osteopathic Medicine (with Temple University)
   University of South Florida
   St. Louis University
   Texas College of Osteopathic Medicine
   Tufts University (Massachusetts)
   Tulane University (Louisianna)

If you'd like your own copy, these publications can be ordered directly by contacting the organizations below:

Association of American Medical Colleges
Publication Orders
2450 N Street, NW
Washington, DC 20037
(202) 828-0416
http://www.aamc.org

American Association of Colleges of Osteopathic Medicine
5550 Friendship Boulevard, Suite 310
Chevy Chase, MD 20815-7231
Main: (301) 968-4100
http://www.aacom.org

Other Selection Factors

• **State residency.** Obviously, everyone knows that attending their state medical school is usually the least expensive option in terms of tuition. But state medical schools also give strong preference to residents of the state. Thus, it behooves every premed student to apply to his or her state medical school(s). Conversely, many state schools accept very few out-of-state applicants. Some schools set strict academic cutoffs for out-of-state applicants, and others accept only the truly gifted or unique out-of-state applicant. If you do not fall into the "truly gifted out-of-state" category, you will save time and money by not wasting your application to a school in a state where you don't reside.

The same goes for Canadian medical schools. They rarely accept non-Canadian medical students. However, they are an option for some students. As stated before, carefully investigate and research any school before you apply.

• **Pass/fail versus A through F.** Some schools continue to use traditional letter grading for every course in their curriculum. Other schools, realizing that basic medical competencies are either achieved or not achieved, have completely switched to a pure pass/fail grading system. Still others, in an attempt to decrease letter grade-induced competition, have established a bizarre pass/fail system consisting of honors, high pass, pass, low pass, and fail. It's hard to imagine the significant difference between this last system and a standard A through F system. A few schools have gone so far as to give letter grades for some courses and pass/fail grades for others. The permutations go on and on.

There is an advantage to a traditional letter grading system. If you graduate from a school without significant prestige or a reputation, having a slew of As on your transcript will place you in the upper echelon of all graduates, regardless of school. On the other hand, a transcript stating that you "merely" passed all your courses will do you no good.

Not much weight should be given to the differences between grading systems. But if you're gunning for a competitive specialty and have the brains to compete for stellar grades, some type of five-scale grading system will probably benefit you. If you're simply looking for a good education without regard to grade differentiation between you and the person sitting next to you in class, seek out the pure pass/fail schools.

• **Combined B.S./M.D. programs.** There still exist numerous programs that combine undergraduate college study with medical school. Some programs simply combine two courses of study, creating an eight-year integrated curriculum. Others tack on the bare-minimum undergraduate science requirements before a full medical school curriculum.

Although the prospect of guaranteed admission to medical school is attractive to many, any program that decreases the time spent in undergraduate college studies should be discouraged. There is something to be said for a mature physician, one who has completed a formal course of study leading to a baccalaureate degree separate from the professional medical degree. To realize a satisfying undergraduate education, all physicians should undergo college studies, not as a pesky medical school prerequisite, but as a formal opportunity for a rich educational experience.

Egregious Error: A student of mine from the Baltimore suburbs once told me that he wanted to attend Johns Hopkins Medical School. When I asked why, he said, "I'm interested in trauma surgery, and Hopkins has their Shock Trauma Center."

When I told him that the Maryland Institute for Emergency Medical Services (MIEMS), commonly known in Maryland as "Shock Trauma," is a prominent part of the University of Maryland Medical Center, across town and distinctly separate from Hopkins, he didn't believe me at first. He thought, "How could a premier trauma center not be associated with the city's most prestigious medical school?"

Imagine what would've happened if he'd actually interviewed at Hopkins and asked about "their Shock Trauma Center"? Never assume anything. Research your schools.

10 Truly Unique Programs

As mentioned previously, every medical school nowadays is touting its modern curriculum changes. Many schools have numerous "tracks" designed to promote their trendy curricula. However, a name alone does not create a truly innovative program. The following schools, on the other hand, have developed significant programs that are more than mere advertisements of the simple innovations mentioned earlier. Instead, these schools have programs that have earned them some form of distinction and truly set them apart. Medical school curricula are rarely set in stone, and changes may occur over time. The following information is the most up-to-date at the time of publication. However, you should always take time to research your schools of interest and their unique programs.

- **Allegheny University of the Health Sciences.** When the Medical College of Pennsylvania and Hahnemann merged, the curricula changed drastically. Students may now voluntarily enter the Program for Integrated Learning, a true problem-based learning track that is offered in lieu of the standard medical curriculum.

- **Brown University.** Brown's Program in Liberal Medical Education is an eight-year continuum encompassing both an undergraduate major course of study and the medical education curriculum. By incorporating these two segments together, students complete their academic training as a whole unit spanning eight years. Brown's program accepts only high school students. Few opportunities exist in exceptional circumstances for students to be admitted directly into the medical school.

- **Case Western Reserve University.** This prestigious school is known for its fondness for "bent-arrow" students as well as for its curricular innovations, which began before anyone heard of "problem-based learning." Their new primary care track requires students to complete their entire third year in a single hospital, with at least one-half of the time spent in an ambulatory setting. Students also see patients in a longitudinal continuity clinic throughout their clinical years. Primary care track students also complete a one-month health policy clerkship and electives tailored to their "personal learning plan."

- **Drew/UCLA Joint Medical Program.** Each year, nearly 25 students are selected for this program, which is designed to train students with a particular interest in serving the urban underserved. This program evolved from the Watts riots in the late 1960s and is one of the true success stories in the continuing effort to provide medical care to underserved populations. Students spend their first two years at the UCLA campus, then spend their clinical years at the Drew campus in Watts. If your interest is in urban primary care for underserved populations, you should seriously consider the Drew program. This program has a separate address:

Drew/UCLA Joint Medical Program
Drew University of Medicine and Science
1621 East 120th Street
Los Angeles, CA 90059
(213) 563-4952

- **Duke University School of Medicine.** At Duke, students complete their basic science training in their first 11 months (!), leaving the second year for required clinical clerkships and the third and fourth years for electives in both the basic sciences and clinical rotations. This curriculum thus allows maximum flexibility for students to pursue their individual interests, experience research opportunities, and delve into the basic sciences concurrently with clinical rotations.

- **East Tennessee State University.** The James H. Quillen College of Medicine has a Rural Primary Care Track, which was developed in conjunction with the W. K. Kellogg Foundation's Community Partnership Program. In this track, students are provided significant exposure to rural primary care medicine in Tennessee with an interdisciplinary (nurse practitioners, physician assistants, etc.) team of practitioners. If rural primary care is your career goal, East Tennessee's program may be just what you're looking for.

• **UC San Francisco—UC Berkeley Joint Medical Program.** Up to 12 students each year are selected to spend three years at Berkeley studying the basic sciences, introductory clinical courses, and a course of study in the social sciences related to medicine. Students then complete their two-year clinical training at UCSF. They are awarded both an M.S. and M.D. degree after completing their studies. This program creates a small society of academic clinicians dedicated to addressing medical problems through various disciplines. This program has a separate address:

UCSF-Berkeley Joint Medical Program, Graduate Office
Health and Medical Sciences Program
570 University Hall #1190
University of California
Berkeley, CA 94720
(510) 642-5671

• **Howard University.** Howard is the first of the nation's three historically black medical schools. Located in Washington, D.C., Howard actively seeks qualified minority applicants to ensure a diverse student body. If you are a minority student and you are looking for a diverse atmosphere, this may be the school for you.

• **The Johns Hopkins University School of Medicine.** Hopkins has a flexible medical admissions program (FlexMed), which allows highly qualified students with guaranteed admissions during their junior year of college so that they can pursue and complete their individual academic, work, or research programs before beginning medical school. In addition, seniors may be offered up to a three-year matriculation deferral to pursue their interests, such as international fellowships, humanitarian service, and work experiences prior to starting medical school.

• **Loma Linda University School of Medicine.** This medical school is owned and operated by the Seventh-Day Adventist Church. The admissions committee readily admits that it gives strong preference to members of the Seventh-Day Adventist Church and nonmembers with strong Christian values. If this describes you and you're interested in combining your faith with your medical practice, Loma Linda may provide a distinct atmosphere that you'll enjoy.

• **Mayo Medical School.** In the third year of school, every student must complete a four-month research project with a faculty member at the Mayo Clinic. It is unusual for a school to require such a long-term biomedical research project of all its students, but if you're interested in research, Mayo will afford this opportunity to all its students.

• **University of Maryland.** The new curriculum at Maryland requires every student to participate in a half-day primary care clinic each week throughout the two clinical years. Just as physicians do in residency, students will scrub out of surgery to see their primary care patients in their clinic one afternoon a week. One of the fundamental aspects of primary care is longitudinal care of your patients. This curricular innovation allows you to follow your patients for two entire years during medical school. This may be one of the best ways to prepare for a primary care career.

• **Meharry Medical College.** Along with Howard and Morehouse, Meharry is one of three historically black medical schools. Located in Tennessee, the school actively seeks qualified minority applicants to ensure a diverse student body. If you prefer the atmosphere of a medical school that seeks such a diverse class, Meharry may suit you.

• **Mercer University School of Medicine.** In addition to the standard curriculum, Mercer has a Community Science Program that pairs students with primary care physicians in rural Georgia, thus providing them with firsthand experience in community health. This track runs throughout the four-year curriculum and culminates with a required rural clerkship in the fourth year. This track was clearly designed for the student with a strong interest in rural primary care.

• **Morehouse School of Medicine.** Morehouse is one of the nation's three historically black medical schools, along with Howard and Meharry. Located in Atlanta, Georgia, Morehouse has a strong tradition of training minority physicians and thus actively seeks qualified minority applicants to create a diverse student body.

• **New Mexico School of Medicine.** There is no distinction between the traditional basic science courses and clinical rotations at New Mexico. In fact, both required clerkships and basic science courses are taught in tandem throughout the first three years. First-year New Mexico students complete rotations typically available only to third-year students from other schools. Students take Step 1 of the Boards at the end of their third year, when all their required coursework is completed. The fourth year is spent with basic science and clinical electives of interest to each student.

- **Ohio State University.** In addition to the traditional educational format, OSU students can participate in the Independent Study Pathway (ISP) or the Problem-Based Learning (PBL) pathway. The ISP provides students with a highly structured objectives guide, leaving the bulk of learning up to the student by use of various computer, library, and faculty resources. The PBL is a true standard PBL track with groups of seven students meeting to review patient cases and problems several times a week.

- **Southern Illinois University School of Medicine.** At SIU, students have the option of selecting the Problem-Based Learning Curriculum (PBLC) for their first two years. This is one of the few true PBL tracks in which groups of five to seven students experience patient cases via computer and standardized patients, then research, study, and learn the material pertinent to the case. The students are self-directed and meet with a faculty tutor to assist in their guided learning.

- **Stanford University School of Medicine.** In the Stanford curriculum, which encourages individuality and intellectual diversity, students are encouraged to take five or six years to complete their M.D. requirements. The standard coursework required of an M.D. is easily supplemented with courses throughout the university, such as literature, sociology, and music. In addition, students are given complete freedom to schedule their courses and clinical rotations to facilitate self-directed learning through research projects, additional degrees, community service, and teaching.

- **Uniformed Service University of the Health Sciences.** USUHS is a federally chartered medical school designed to train physicians for the Armed Services and the Public Health Service. Tuition is free (yes, free!), but graduates are required to serve for a number of years as physicians in their selected military branch or in the Public Health Service. Students cannot be more than 30 years of age on June 30 of the year of matriculation. If you are planning a military or Public Health Service career, you should seriously consider USUHS.

• **Yale University.** No grades. That's right, no grades at all. Yale believes that medical students should develop their maturity and responsibility throughout their curriculum, so exams are anonymous, and independent study and research are encouraged in this highly flexible curriculum. How do Yale grads compete without grades? They are subjectively assessed by the faculty and receive written evaluations describing their work.

11 How Many Applications?

This is a perennial question for many premed students. Surely you should not apply to every single medical school out there. Nor should you apply only to two or three prestigious medical schools alone. What's the in-between balance? Studies have shown that your chances of admission actually decline after 20 applications. But there are numerous variables to consider when making your decision. Here are some handy guidelines.

• **Apply to your state school(s).** Since you automatically have a preferential chance of admission at your state school, you must automatically apply each of your state medical schools. For students in the larger states, this amounts to many schools, but unless you have extreme reservations about attending a particular school, you should stack the deck in your favor. Also, some schools are not obviously state supported, yet still provide preferential consideration for state residents (e.g., University of Pittsburgh and University of Pennsylvania).

Some states, such as some in New England, Alaska, and other Western states, have no state medical school. However, they typically have reciprocal preference with other states, and thus, students in these states have preferential consideration at other states' schools. These preferences are not always obvious (e.g., Delaware residents have preference at Thomas Jefferson University; Idaho residents have preference in Washington State). **Investigate where you are given preferential admissions, and apply there.**

• **Location, location, location.** Many students prefer living in a particular region of the country or in a particular city because of family or for other reasons. Thus, it is obvious that you would apply to several medical schools in that area. Don't hesitate to cluster your applications, and frankly admit that you prefer that region of the country. However, don't expect your personal preference to carry any more weight with the admissions committee. And again, research your schools. Remember the first "Egregious Error" described in Chapter 9.

• **Money talks.** Each medical school application costs money—lots of it. The number of schools you apply to may be limited by the amount you have to spend on primary as well as secondary applications. Choose carefully.

Unfortunately, medical school tuition is very pricey. Again, your state school probably has the least expensive tuition for you. But you must also consider living expenses and other costs associated with moving to another location. Once again, the third book in this series, *The Right Price,* is a good source for all that you must consider when figuring the costs of medical school. If certain schools are prohibitively expensive for you, then don't bother applying there. Of course, as a medical student you will have absolutely no problem finding an adequate number of loans to cover all your expenses. However, there's no guarantee that these loans will carry a reasonable interest rate.

Never assume that a higher tuition necessarily implies a higher quality of education. In fact, when comparing schools with radically different tuitions (usually your state school vs. any other school), you should always ask yourself, "What am I getting for the additional thousands of dollars that this school costs compared with another?"

It never hurts to research your financial aid options and the amount of grants and scholarships (i.e., funds that don't need to be paid back) available at certain schools. Some schools have special programs that significantly reduce tuition (e.g., Mayo Medical School and the University of Pennsylvania) and deserve investigating. Again, research your schools.

• **Match your interests to schools.** The previous chapter provided information on schools with truly unique and innovative curricula designed to encourage and develop particular interests or medical careers. You should investigate several schools that match your career interests and apply to them. Obviously, your application should promote your particular interest in their special programs. Again, the key to success is to research your medical schools. It makes no sense to apply to schools with strong primary care programs if you're interested in a subspecialty, and vice versa. **Research your schools.**

• **Variety is the spice of applications.** Although few schools stand out with unique curricula that may match your interests, all schools have peculiarities that make them minimally discernible from other schools. If your entire application list consists of schools that are similar to each other and if you are not suitable for one school, chances are you won't be admitted to any of the rest either. You should seek a balance with several different types of schools that vary by location, state affiliation, unique programs, and interests that match your own. In other words, don't apply only to the Ivy League schools or only to M.D.-Ph.D. programs. Nor should you apply only to "safety schools." Spread yourself out, take a few chances, but always be reasonable.

12 U.S. and Canadian Medical Schools

Following is a complete address and phone list of U.S. and Canadian medical schools. Select the ones that interest you, look up their web pages on the Internet, and contact them to ask for the latest catalog or speak with the admissions director. The best way to obtain accurate information about individual programs is to get it directly from the source. (PUBLISHER'S NOTE: To the best of our knowledge, mailing addresses, phone numbers, e-mail addresses, and Website addresses are correct, but this information—especially Website addresses, e-mail addresses, and telephone area codes—may change over time.)

Alabama

University of Alabama School of Medicine
Office of Admissions, VH100
Birmingham, AL 35294-0019
(205) 934-2330
E-mail: jellison@uasom.meis.uab.edu
http://www.uab.edu

University of South Alabama College of Medicine
Office of Admissions, 2015 MSB
Mobile, AL 36688-0002
(334) 460-7176
http://www.usouthal.edu

Arizona

Arizona College of Osteopathic Medicine
Midwestern University
Office of Admissions, AZCOM
19555 N. 59th Avenue
Glendale, AZ 85308
(888) 247-9277 or (602) 572-3215
http://www.aacom.org/acom.htm

University of Arizona College of Medicine
Admissions Office, Room 2209
P. O. Box 245075
Tucson, AZ 85724-5075
(520) 626-6214
http://www.medicine.arizona.edu

Arkansas

University of Arkansas College of Medicine
Office of Student Admissions, Slot 551
4301 West Markham Street
Little Rock, AR 72205-7199
(501) 686-5354
E-mail: SouthTomG@Exchange.uams.edu
http://www.uams.edu/com

California

San Francisco College of Osteopathic Medicine
1210 Scott Street
San Francisco, California 94115
(888) 880-SFDO (in California); (888) 887-SFDO (outside California);
    (415) 292-0407
http://www.aacom.org/sfcom.htm

Loma Linda University School of Medicine
Associate Dean for Admissions
Loma Linda, CA 92350
(800) 422-4558 or (909) 824-4467
http://www.llu.edu

Stanford University School of Medicine
Office of Admissions
851 Welch Road, Room 154
Palo Alto, CA 94304-1677
(650) 723-6861
http://med-www.stanford.edu

University of California—Davis, School of Medicine
Office of Admissions
One Shields Avenue
Davis, CA 95616
(530) 752-2717
http://www-med.ucdavis.edu

University of California—Irvine, College of Medicine
Medical Education Building, 802
Irvine, CA 92717
(800) 824-5388
http://www.com.uci.edu

University of California—Los Angeles, School of Medicine
Office of Admissions
12-105 Center for Health Sciences
Box 957035
10833 LeConte Avenue
Los Angeles, CA 90095-7035
(310) 825-6081
http://www.medsch.ucla.edu

Drew/UCLA Joint Medical Program
Drew University of Medicine and Science
1621 East 120th Street
Los Angeles, CA 90059
(213) 563-4952
http://www.cdrewu.edu

University of California—San Diego, School of Medicine
Office of Admissions, 0621
Medical Teaching Facility
9500 Gilman Drive
La Jolla, CA 92093-0621
(619) 534-3880
http://medicine.ucsd.edu

University of California—San Francisco, School of Medicine
Admissions, C—200, Box 0408
San Francisco, CA 94143
(415) 476-4044
http://www.som.ucsf.edu

UCSF-Berkeley Joint Medical Program
Graduate Office
Health and Medical Sciences Program
570 University Hall #1190
University of California
Berkeley, CA 94720
(510) 642-5671
http://violet.berkeley.edu/jmp-hms/jmphmpg.html

University of Southern California, School of Medicine
Admission Office
1975 Zonal Avenue
KAM 100C
Los Angeles, CA 90033
(323) 442-2552
E-mail: medadmit@hsc.usc.edu
http://www.usc.edu/schools/medicine

Western University of the Health Sciences
College of Osteopathic Medicine of the Pacific
Office of Admissions
309 E. Second Street
College Plaza
Pomona, California 91766-1889
(909) 623-6116
http://www.westernu.edu/comp.html

Colorado
University of Colorado School of Medicine
Medical School Admissions
4200 East 9th Avenue, C-297
Denver, CO 80262
(303) 315-7361
http://www.uchsc.edu

Connecticut

University of Connecticut School of Medicine
Office of Admissions and Student Affairs
263 Farmington Avenue, Rm. AG-031
Farmington, CT 06030-1905
(860) 679-4713
E-mail: sargis@nso1.uchc.edu
http://www9.uchc.edu/index.html

Yale University School of Medicine
Office of Admissions
367 Cedar Street
New Haven, CT 06510
(860) 785-2696
E-mail: medicalschool.admissions@quickmail.yale.edu
http://info.med.yale.edu/medical/

District of Columbia

George Washington University School of Medicine and Health Sciences
Office of Admissions
2300 Eye Street, NW, Room 615
Washington, DC 20037
(202) 994-3506
E-mail: medadmit@gwunix2.gwu.edu
http://www.gwumc.edu

Georgetown University School of Medicine
Office of Admissions
3900 Reservoir Road, NW
Washington, DC 20007
(202) 687-1154
http://www.dml.georgetown.edu/schmed

Howard University College of Medicine
Admissions Office
520 W Street, NW
Washington, DC 20059
(202) 806-6270
http://www.med.howard.edu

Florida

Florida State University Program in Medical Sciences
104 SCN
Tallahassee, FL 32306-4300
(850) 644-1855
http://www.fsu.edu/~pims/pims.html

Nova Southeastern University College of Osteopathic Medicine
Admissions Office
3200 S. University Drive
Ft. Lauderdale, Florida 33328
(954) 262-1101 or (800) 356-0026
E-mail: rogeria@hpd.nova.edu
http://medicine.nova.edu

University of Florida College of Medicine
Chair, Medical Selection Committee
J. Hillis Miller Health Center
P.O. Box 100216
Gainesville, FL 32610
(904) 392-4569
http://www.med.ufl.edu

University of Miami School of Medicine
Office of Admissions
P.O. Box 016159 (R-159)
Miami, FL 33101
(305) 243-6791
E-mail: miami-md@mednet.med.miami.edu
http://www.med.miami.edu

University of South Florida College of Medicine
Office of Admissions, Box 3
12901 Bruce B. Downs Blvd.
Tampa, FL 33612-4799
(813) 974-2229
http://com1.med.usf.edu

Georgia

Emory University School of Medicine
Medical School Admissions
Emory University School of Medicine
303 Woodruff Health Sciences Center Administration Building
1440 Clifton Road, NE
Atlanta, GA 30322-4510
(404) 727-5660
E-mail: medschadmiss@medadm.emory.edu
http://www.emory.edu/WHSC/MED

Medical College of Georgia School of Medicine
Associate Dean for Admissions
AA-2040
Augusta, Georgia 30912-4760
(706) 721-3186
E-mail: sclmed.stdadmin@mail.mcg.edu
http://www.mcg.edu

Mercer University School of Medicine
Office of Admissions and Student Affairs
1550 College Street
Macon, GA 31207
(912) 752-2542
E-mail: kothanek_je@mercer.edu
http://musm.mercer.edu

Morehouse School of Medicine
Admissions and Student Affairs
720 Westview Drive, SW
Atlanta, GA 30310-1495
(404) 752-1650
http://www.msm.edu

Hawaii

University of Hawaii, John A. Burns School of Medicine
Office of Admissions
1960 East—West Road
Honolulu, HI 96822
(808) 956-8300
E-mail: nishikim@jabsom.biomed.hawaii.edu
http://medworld.biomed.hawaii.edu

Illinois

Chicago College of Osteopathic Medicine
Midwestern University (CCOM)
Office of Admissions
CCOM Midwestern University
555 31st Street
Downers Grove, IL 60515
(800) 458-6253 or (630) 969-4400
http://www.midwestern.edu/Pages/CCOM.html

Chicago Medical School, Finch University of Health Sciences
Office of Admissions
3333 Green Bay Road
North Chicago, IL 60064-3095
(847) 578-3205
E-mail: jonesk@mis.finchms.edu
http://www.finchcms.edu

University of Chicago, Pritzker School of Medicine
Office of the Dean of Students
924 East 57th Street, BLSC 104
Chicago, IL 60637
(773) 702-1939
http://pritzker.bsd.uchicago.edu

University of Illinois College of Medicine
Office of Medical College Admissions
Room 165 CME M/C 783
808 South Wood Street
Chicago, IL 60612-7302
(312) 996-5635
http://www.uic.edu/depts/mcam

Stritch School of Medicine
Loyola University of Chicago
Office of Admissions, Room 1752
2160 South First Avenue
Maywood, IL 60153
(708) 216-3229
http://www.meddean.luc.edu/

Northwestern University Medical School
Associate Dean for Admissions
Morton Building 1-606
303 East Chicago Avenue
Chicago, IL 60611-3008
(312) 503-8206
http://www.nums.nwu.edu

Rush Medical College
Office of Admissions
524 Academic Facility
600 South Paulina Street
Chicago, IL 60612
(312) 942-6913
E-mail: medcol@rush.edu
http://www.rushu.rush.edu/medcol

Southern Illinois University School of Medicine
Office of Student Affairs
P.O. Box 19230
Springfield, IL 62794-1226
(217) 782-2860
http://www.siumed.edu

Indiana

Indiana University School of Medicine
Medical School Admissions Office
Fesler Hall 213
1120 South Drive
Indianapolis, IN 46202-5113
(317) 274-3772
http://www.medicine.iu.edu/home.html

Iowa

University of Iowa College of Medicine
Director of Admissions
100 Medicine Administration Building
Iowa City, IA 52242-1101
(319) 335-8052
E-mail: medical-admissions@uiowa.edu
http://www.medicine.uiowa.edu/

University of Osteopathic Medicine and Health Sciences
College of Osteopathic Medicine and Surgery
Dennis L. Bates, Ph.D.
Director of Admissions and Financial Aid
3200 Grand Avenue
Des Moines, Iowa 50312
(515) 271-1450 or (800) 240-2767, ext. 1450.
E-mail: DOadmit@uomhs.edu
http://www.uomhs.edu

Kansas

University of Kansas School of Medicine
Associate Dean for Admissions
3901 Rainbow Blvd.
Kansas City, KS 66160-7301
(913) 588-5245
http://www.kumc.edu

Kentucky

Pikeville College School of Osteopathic Medicine
214 Sycamore St.
Pikeville, KY 41501
(606) 432-9640
http://pcsom.pc.edu/

University of Kentucky College of Medicine
Admissions, Room MN-102
Office of Education
Chandler Medical Center
800 Rose Street
Lexington, KY 40536-0084
(606) 323-6161
http://www.comed.uky.edu

University of Louisville School of Medicine
Medicine-Admissions Office
University of Louisville
Abell Administration Center
323 East Chestnut Street
Louisville, KY 40202-3866
(800) 334-8635, ext. 5193 or (502) 852-5193
http://www.louisville.edu/medschool

Louisiana

Louisiana State University—New Orleans, School of Medicine
Admissions Office
1901 Perdido Street, Box P3-4
New Orleans, LA 70112-1393
(504) 568-6262
http://www.medschool.lsumc.edu

Louisiana State University—Shreveport, School of Medicine
Office of Student Admissions
P.O. Box 33932
Shreveport, LA 71130-3932
(318) 675-5190
E-mail: shvadm@lsumc.edu
http://www.sh.lsumc.edu

Tulane University School of Medicine
Office of Admissions
1430 Tulane Ave, SL67
New Orleans, LA 70112-2699
(504) 588-5187
E-mail: medsch@tmcpop.tmc.tulane.edu
http://www.mcl.tulane.edu

Maine

University of New England College of Osteopathic Medicine
Admissions Office
11 Hills Beach Road
Biddeford, ME 04005-9599
(800) 477-4UNE or 207-283-0171 ext. 2297
http://www.une.edu/COM/compage1.html

Maryland

Johns Hopkins University School of Medicine
Committee on Admission
720 Rutland Avenue
Baltimore, MD 21205-2196
(410) 955-3182
http://infonet.welch.jhu.edu

University of Maryland School of Medicine
Committee on Admissions, Room 1-005
655 West Baltimore Street
Baltimore, MD 21201
(410) 706-7478
http://som1.umaryland.edu

Uniformed Services University of the Health Sciences
F. Edward Hebert School of Medicine
Admissions Office, Room A-1041
4301 Jones Bridge Road
Bethesda, MD 20814-4799
(800) 772-1743
http://www.usuhs.mil

Massachusetts

Boston University School of Medicine
Admissions Office
715 Albany Street L-124
Boston, MA 02118
(617) 638-4630
http://www.bumc.bu.edu

Harvard Medical School
Office of Admissions
25 Shattuck Street
Boston, MA 02115-6092
(617) 432-1550
E-mail: HMSADM@warren.med.harvard.edu
http://www.med.harvard.edu

University of Massachusetts Medical School
Associate Dean for Admissions
55 Lake Avenue, North
Worcester, MA 01655
(508) 856-2323
E-mail: Admissions@banyan.ummed.edu
http://www.ummed.edu

Tufts University School of Medicine
Office of Admissions
136 Harrison Avenue
Boston, MA 02111
(617) 636-6571
http://www.tufts.edu/med

Michigan

University of Michigan Medical School
Admissions Office
M4130 Medical Science Building I
1301 Catherine
Ann Arbor, MI 48109-0624
(734) 764-6317
http://www.med.umich.edu/medschool

Michigan State University College of Human Medicine
Office of Admissions
A-239 Life Sciences
East Lansing, MI 48824-1317
(517) 353-9620
E-mail: MDAdmissions@msu.edu
http://www.chm.msu.edu

Michigan State University College of Osteopathic Medicine
Director of Admissions
C110 East Fee Hall
East Lansing, MI 48824-1316
(517) 353-7740
http://www.com.msu.edu

Wayne State University School of Medicine
Director of Admissions
540 East Canfield, Room 1310
Detroit, MI 48201
(313) 577-1466
http://www.phypc.med.wayne.edu

Minnesota

Mayo Medical School
Admissions Committee
200 First Street, SW
Rochester, MN 55905
(507) 284-3671
http://www.mayo.edu/mms

University of Minnesota—Duluth, School of Medicine
Office of Admissions, Room 180
10 University Drive
Duluth, MN 55812
(218) 726-8511
E-mail: jcarls10@d.umn.edu
http://www.d.umn.edu/medweb

University of Minnesota Medical School
Office of Admissions and Student Affairs
Box 293—UMHC, 3-100 Owre Hall
420 Delaware Street, SE
Minneapolis, MN 55455-0310
(612) 624-1188
http://www.med.umn.edu

Mississippi

University of Mississippi School of Medicine
Chair, Admissions Committee
2500 North State Street
Jackson, MS 39216-4505
(601) 984-5010
http://umc.edu/medicine

Missouri

Kirksville College of Osteopathic Medicine
Office of Admissions
800 West Jefferson
Kirksville, MO 63501
(816) 626-2237 or (800) 626-5266 ext. 2237
http://www.kcom.edu

University of Missouri—Columbia, School of Medicine
Office of Admissions
MA202 Medical Sciences Bldg.
One Hospital Drive
Columbia, MO 65212
(573) 882-2923
E-mail: shari_l._swindell@muccmail.missouri.edu
http://www.hsc.missouri.edu/medicine

University of Missouri—Kansas City, School of Medicine
Council on Selection
2411 Holmes
Kansas City, MO 64108-2792
(816) 235-1808
http://research.med.umkc.edu

St. Louis University School of Medicine
Admissions Committee
1402 South Grand Blvd.
St. Louis, MO 63104
(314) 577-8205
E-mail: medadmis@slu.edu
http://www.slu.edu/colleges/med

University of Health Sciences, College of Osteopathic Medicine
Office of Admissions
1750 Independence Avenue
Kansas City, Missouri 64106-1453
(800) 234-4UHS, ext. 847
http://www.uhs.edu

Washington University School of Medicine
Office of Admissions
660 South Euclid Avenue, #8107
St. Louis, MO 63110
(314) 362-6858
E-mail: wumscoa@molly.wustl.edu
http://medinfo.wustl.edu

Nebraska

Creighton University School of Medicine
Office of Admissions
2500 California Plaza
Omaha, NE 68178
(402) 280-2798
http://medicine.creighton.edu

University of Nebraska College of Medicine
Office of Academic and Student Affairs
986585 Nebraska Medical Center
Omaha NE 68198-6585
http://www.unmc.edu/UNCOM

Nevada

University of Nevada School of Medicine
Office of Admissions and Student Affairs
Manville Medical Building/357
Reno, NV 89557-0046
(775) 784-6063
http://www.unr.edu/med

New Hampshire

Dartmouth Medical School
Admissions
7020 Remsen, Room 306
Hanover, NH 03755-3833
(603) 650-1505
http://www.dartmouth.edu/dms

New Jersey

UMDNJ—New Jersey Medical School
Director of Admissions
185 South Orange Avenue
Newark, NJ 07103-2714
(973) 972-4631
http://www.umdnj.edu/njmsweb

UMDNJ—R. W. Johnson Medical School
Office of Admissions
675 Hoes Lane
Piscataway, NJ 08854-5635
(732) 235-4576
http://www2.umdnj.edu/rwjpweb

UMDNJ—School of Osteopathic Medicine
Admissions Office
Academic Center
One Medical Center Drive, Suite 162A
Stratford, NJ 08084
(609) 566-7050
http://www3.umdnj.edu/som/index.html

New Mexico

University of New Mexico School of Medicine
Office of Admissions and Student Affairs
Basic Medical Sciences Building, Room 107
Albuquerque, NM 87131-5166
(505) 272-4766
http://hsc.unm.edu/som/

New York

Albany Medical College
Office of Admissions
47 New Scotland Avenue, Mail Code 3
Albany, NY 12208
(518) 262-5521
http://www.amc.edu

Albert Einstein College of Medicine
Office of Admissions
Jack and Pearl Resnick Campus
1300 Morris Park Avenue
Bronx, NY 10461
(718) 430-2106

Columbia University, College of Physicians and Surgeons
Office of Admissions, Room 1-416
630 West 168th Street
New York, NY 10032
(212) 305-3595
http://cpmcnet.columbia.edu/dept/ps

Mount Sinai School of Medicine
Director of Admissions
Annenberg Bldg., Room 5-04
One Gustave L. Levy Place, Box 1002
New York, NY 10029-6574
(212) 241-6696
http://www.mssm.edu

New York College of Osteopathic Medicine
New York Institute of Technology
Director of Admissions
Old Westbury, NY 11568
(516) 626-6947
http://www.nyit.edu

New York Medical College
Office of Admissions
Room 127, Sunshine Cottage
Valhalla, NY 10595
(914) 594-4510
http://www.nymc.edu

New York University School of Medicine
Admissions Office
550 First Avenue
New York, NY 10016
(212) 263-5290
http://www.med.nyu.edu/som/index.html

University of Rochester School of Medicine and Dentistry
Director of Admissions
Medical Center Box 601
Rochester, NY 14642-8601
(716) 275-4539
E-mail: mdadmish@urmc.rochester.edu
http://www.urmc.rochester.edu/SMD

SUNY—Brooklyn, College of Medicine
Director of Admissions
450 Clarkson Avenue, Box 60M
Brooklyn, NY 11203-2098
(718) 270-2446
http://md.hscbklyn.edu/

SUNY—Buffalo, School of Medicine
Office of Medical Admissions
40 Biomedical Education Building
3435 Main Street
Buffalo, NY 14214-3013
(716) 829-3467
E-mail: jjrosso@acsu.buffalo.edu
http://www.smbs.buffalo.edu

SUNY—Stony Brook, School of Medicine
Health Sciences Center
Committee on Admissions
Level 4, Room 147
Stony Brook, NY 11794-8434
(516) 444-2113
E-mail: admissions@dean.som.sunysb.edu
http://www.uhmc.sunysb.edu/som

SUNY—Syracuse, College of Medicine
Admissions Office
CAB Room 204
155 Elizabeth Blackwell Street
Syracuse, NY 13210
(315) 464-4570
E-mail: admiss@hscsyr.edu
http://www.hscsyr.edu/home/medicine

Weill Medical College of Cornell University
Office of Admissions
445 East 69th Street
New York, NY 10021
(212) 746-6565
http://www.med.cornell.edu

North Carolina

Wake Forest University School of Medicine
Office of Medical School Admissions
Medical Center Blvd.
Winston-Salem, NC 27157-1090
(336) 716-4264
http://isnet.is.wfu.edu/education/admissions

Duke University School of Medicine
Committee on Admissions
Box 3710 Medical Center
Durham, NC 27710
(919) 684-2985
http://www2.mc.duke.edu/som

East Carolina University School of Medicine
Assistant Dean, Office of Admissions
Greenville, NC 27858-4354
(919) 816-2202
http://www.med.ecu.edu

University of North Carolina at Chapel Hill, School of Medicine
Admissions Office
CB# 7000 MacNider Hall
Chapel Hill, NC 27599-7000
(919) 962-8331
E-mail: esmann@med.unc.edu
http://www.med.unc.edu

North Dakota

University of North Dakota School of Medicine
Secretary, Committee on Admissions
501 North Columbia Road, Box 9037
Grand Forks, ND 58202-9037
(701) 777-4221
E-mail: judy.heit@medicine.und.nodak.edu
http://www.med.und.nodak.edu

Ohio

Case Western Reserve University School of Medicine
Associate Dean for Admissions
10900 Euclid Avenue
Cleveland, OH 44106-4920
(216) 368-3450
http://www.cwru.edu

University of Cincinnati College of Medicine
Office of Student Affairs/Admissions
P.O. Box 670552
Cincinnati, OH 45267-0552
(513) 558-7314
http://www.med.uc.edu

Medical College of Ohio
Admissions Office
P.O. Box 10008
Toledo, OH 43699
(419) 383-4229
http://www.mco.edu

Northeastern Ohio Universities College of Medicine
Office of Admissions and Educational Research
P.O. Box 95
Rootstown, OH 44272-0095
(216) 325-2511
E-mail: admission@neoucom.edu
http://www.neoucom.edu

Ohio State University College of Medicine and Public Health
Admissions Committee
270-A Meiling Hall
370 West Ninth Avenue
Columbus, OH 43210-1238
(614) 292-7137
E-mail: admiss-med@osu.edu
http://www.med.ohio-state.edu

Ohio University College of Osteopathic Medicine
Office of Admissions
102 Grosvenor Hall
Athens, OH 45701-2979
1-800-345-1560
http://www.ohiou.edu

Wright State University School of Medicine
Office of Student Affairs/Admissions
P.O. Box 1751
Dayton, OH 45401
(937) 775-2934
E-mail: som_saa@wright.edu
http://www.med.wright.edu

Oklahoma

University of Oklahoma College of Medicine
Office of Admissions, BMSB 337
P.O. Box 26901
Oklahoma City, OK 73190
(405) 271-2331
E-mail: AdminMed@ouhsc.edu
http://www.uokhsc.edu

Oklahoma State University College of Osteopathic Medicine
Admissions Office
1111 West 17th St
Tulsa, OK 74107-1898
(918) 582-1972 or (800) 677-1972
http://osu.com.okstate.edu/osucom.html

Oregon

Oregon Health Sciences University School of Medicine
Office of Education & Student Affairs, L102
3181 SW Sam Jackson Park Road
Portland, OR 97201
(503) 494-2998
http://www.ohsu.edu/som

Pennsylvania

Allegheny University of the Health Sciences
MCP Hahnemann School of Medicine
Admissions Office
2900 Queen Lane Avenue
Philadelphia, PA 19129
(215) 991-8202
E-mail: admis@ef.allegheny.edu
http://www.auhs.edu

Jefferson Medical College
Associate Dean for Admissions
1025 Walnut Street, Suite 116
Philadelphia, PA 19107-5083
(215) 955-6983
http://jeffline.tju.edu/CWIS/JMC/jmc.html

Lake Erie College of Osteopathic Medicine
Office of Admissions
1858 West Grandview Boulevard
Erie, PA 16509
(814) 866-6641
http://www.lecom.edu

Pennsylvania State University College of Medicine
Office of Student Affairs
P.O. Box 850
Hershey, PA 17033
(717) 531-8755
http://www.collmed.psu.edu

Philadelphia College of Osteopathic Medicine
Assistant Dean for Admissions
4170 City Avenue
Philadelphia, PA 19131
(800) 999-6998
http://www.pcom.edu

University of Pennsylvania School of Medicine
Office of Admissions and Financial Aid
Edward J. Stemmler Hall, Suite 100
3450 Hamilton Walk
Philadelphia, PA 19020
(215) 898-8001
http://www.med.upenn.edu

University of Pittsburgh School of Medicine
Office of Admissions
518 Scaife Hall
Pittsburgh, PA 15261
(412) 648-9891
E-mail: admissions@fs1.dean-med.pitt.edu
http://www.dean-med.pitt.edu

Temple University School of Medicine
Office of Admissions
Suite 305, Student Faculty Center
3340 North Broad Street
Philadelphia, PA 19140
(215) 707-3656
E-mail: gmorton@nimbus.ocis.temple.edu
http://www.temple.edu/medschool

Puerto Rico

Universidad Central Del Caribe, School of Medicine
Office of Admissions
Ramon Ruiz Arnau University Hospital
Call Box 60-327
Bayamon, PR 00960-6032
(787) 740-1611 ext 210

Ponce School of Medicine
Admissions Office
P.O. Box 7004
Ponce, PR 00732
(787) 840-2511

University of Puerto Rico School of Medicine
Central Admissions Office
Medical Sciences Campus
P.O. Box 365067
San Juan, PR 00936-5067
(787) 758-2525 ext 5213
E-mail: r_aponte@rcmad.upr.clu.edu
http://wwwrcm.upr.clu.edu

Rhode Island
Brown University School of Medicine
Office of Admissions and Financial Aid
97 Waterman St., Box G-A212
Providence, RI 02912-9706
(401) 863-2149
E-mail: MedSchool_Admissions@brown.edu
http://biomed.brown.edu/Medicine.html

South Carolina
Medical University of South Carolina, College of Medicine
Office of Enrollment Services
171 Ashley Avenue, Suite 203
P.O. Box 250402
Charleston, SC 29425
(843) 792-3283
E-mail: gravesb@musc.edu
http://www2.musc.edu/medicine.html

University of South Carolina School of Medicine
Dr. Robert F. Sabalis
Medical Education & Academic Affairs
6311 Garner's Ferry Rd.
Columbia, SC 29208
(803) 733-1531
http://www.med.sc.edu

South Dakota
University of South Dakota School of Medicine
Office of Student Affairs, Room 105
1400 W 22nd St.
Sioux Falls, SD 57105
(605) 357-1422
http://www.usd.edu/med

Tennessee
East Tennessee State University, James H. Quillen College of Medicine
Assistant Dean for Admissions and Records
P.O. Box 70580
Johnson City, TN 37614-0580
(423) 439-6221
E-mail: sacom@etsu.edu
http://qcom.etsu.edu

Meharry Medical College School of Medicine
Director, Admissions and Records
1005 Dr. D. B. Todd, Jr. Boulevard
Nashville, TN 37208-3599
(615) 327-6223
http://www.mmc.edu

University of Tennessee College of Medicine
Admissions Office, Room 307
790 Madison Avenue
Memphis, TN 38163-2166
(901) 448-5559
http://utmgopher.utmem.edu

Vanderbilt School of Medicine
Office of Admissions
209 Light Hall
Nashville, TN 37232-0685
(615) 322-2145
E-mail: medsch.admis@mcmail.vanderbilt.edu
http://www.mc.vanderbilt.edu/medschool

Texas

Baylor College of Medicine
Office of Admissions
One Baylor Plaza
Houston, TX 77030
(713) 798-4842
E-mail: melodym@bcm.tmc.edu
http://www.bcm.tmc.edu

Texas A & M University College of Medicine
Assistant Dean for Admissions
Texas A&M University Health Science Center
College of Medicine
Office of Student Affairs and Admissions
159 Joe H. Reynolds Medical Building
College Station, TX 77843-1114
(409) 845-7743
E-mail: med-stu-aff@tamu.edu
http://tamushsc.tamu.edu/COM/COMmain.html

Texas Tech University School of Medicine
Health Sciences Center
Office of Admissions-2B116
Lubbock, TX 79430
(806) 743-2297
http://www.ttuhsc.edu/pages/med.htm

University of North Texas Health Science Center
Texas College of Osteopathic Medicine
Office of Medical Student Admissions
3500 Camp Bowie Boulevard
Fort Worth, TX 76107-2699
(817) 735-2204 or (800) 535-TCOM
http://www.hsc.unt.edu/education/tcom

University of Texas—Galveston, Medical Branch at Galveston
Office of Admissions
G.210, Ashbel Smith Bldg.
Galveston, TX 77555-1317
(409) 772-3517
E-mail: pwylie@mspo4.med.utmb.edu
http://www.utmb.edu

University of Texas—Houston, Medical School at Houston
Office of Admissions, Room G-024
P.O. Box 20708
Houston, TX 77225
(713) 500-5116
http://www.med.uth.tmc.edu

University of Texas—San Antonio, Medical School at San Antonio
Medical School Admissions/Registrar's Office
Health Science Center
7703 Floyd Curl Drive
San Antonio, TX 78284-7701
(210) 567-2665
http://www.uthscsa.edu

University of Texas—Southwestern, Southwestern Medical School
Office of the Registrar
5323 Harry Hines Blvd.
Dallas, TX 75235-9162
(214) 648-5617
http://www.swmed.edu/education/medical

Utah

University of Utah School of Medicine
Director, Medical School Admissions
50 North Medical Drive
Salt Lake City, UT 84132
(801) 581-7498
E-mail: deans.admissions@hsc.utah.edu
http://www.med.utah.edu/som

Vermont

University of Vermont College of Medicine
Admissions Office
C-225 Given Bldg.
Burlington, VT 05405
(802) 656-2154
http://salus.uvm.edu

Virginia

Eastern Virginia Medical School
Office of Admissions
721 Fairfax Avenue
Norfolk, VA 23507-2000
(757) 446-5812
http://www.evms.edu

Medical College of Virginia
Virginia Commonwealth University
Medical School Admissions
P.O. Box 980565
Richmond, VA 23298-0565
(804) 828-9790
http://views.vcu.edu

University of Virginia School of Medicine
Director of Admissions
Box 235
Charlottesville, VA 22908
(804) 924-5571
http://www.med.virginia.edu/schools/medschl.html

Washington

University of Washington School of Medicine
Office of Admissions
Health Sciences Center A-300, Box 356340
Seattle, WA 98195-6340
(206) 543-7212
E-mail: askuwsom@u.washington.edu
http://www.washington.edu/medical/som

West Virginia

Marshall University School of Medicine
Director of Admissions and Student Affairs
1600 Medical Center Drive
Suite 3400
Huntington, WV 25701-3655
(304) 691-1738
http://musom.marshall.edu

West Virginia School of Osteopathic Medicine
Director of Admissions
400 North Lee Street
Lewisburg, WV 24901
(800) 356-7836 (in West Virginia); (800) 537-7077 (outside West Virginia)
http://www.wvsom.edu

West Virginia University School of Medicine
Office of Admissions and Records
Health Sciences Center
P.O. Box 9815
Morgantown, WV 26506
(304) 293-3521
E-mail: dhall@wvuhsc1.hsc.wvu.edu
http://www.hsc.wvu.edu/som

Wisconsin

Medical College of Wisconsin
Office of Admissions and Registrar
8701 Watertown Plank Road
P.O. Box 26509
Milwaukee, WI 53226
(414) 456-8246
http://www.mcw.edu

University of Wisconsin Medical School
Admissions Committee
Medical Sciences Center, Room 1250
1300 University Avenue
Madison, WI 53706
(608) 263-4925
E-mail: Janice.Waisman@mail.admin.wisc.edu
http://www.medsch.wisc.edu/index.html

CANADA

Alberta

University of Alberta
Faculty of Medicine and Oral Health Sciences
Admissions Officer
2-45 Medical Sciences Building
Edmonton, Alberta
Canada T6G 2H7
(403) 492-6350

E-mail: admissions@med.ualberta.ca
http://www.med.ualberta.ca

University of Calgary
Faculty of Medicine
Office of Admissions
3330 Hospital Drive, NW
Calgary, Alberta
Canada T2N 4N1
(403) 220-4262
E-mail: meyers@med.ucalgary.ca
http://www.ucalgary.ca/UofC/faculties/medicine

British Columbia

University of British Columbia
Faculty of Medicine
Office of the Dean, Admissions Office
317-2194 Health Sciences Mall
Vancouver, British Columbia
Canada V6T 1Z3
(604) 822-4482
http://www.med.ubc.ca

Manitoba

University of Manitoba
Registrar, Faculty of Medicine
S204-753 McDermot Avenue
Winnipeg, Manitoba
Canada R3E 0W3
(204) 789-3569
E-mail: registrar_med@cc.umanitoba.ca
http://www.umanitoba.ca/faculties/medicine

Newfoundland

Memorial University of Newfoundland
Admissions Office, Faculty of Medicine
Room 276, Health Sciences Centre
St. John's, Newfoundland
Canada A1B 3V6
(709) 737-6615
E-mail: munmed@morgan.ucs.mun.ca
http://www.med.mun.ca/med

Nova Scotia
  Dalhousie University
  Faculty of Medicine
  Admissions Coordinator
  Room C-132, Lower Level
  Clinical Research Centre
  5849 University Avenue
  Halifax, Nova Scotia
  Canada B3H 4H7
  (902) 494-1083
  http://www.mcms.dal.ca

Ontario
  McMaster University, School of Medicine
  Admissions and Records
  Faculty of Health Sciences
  1200 Main Street West
  Hamilton, Ontario
  Canada L8N 3Z5
  (905) 525-9140, ext. 22114
  E-mail: mdadmit@fhs.csu.mcmaster.ca
  http://www-fhs.mcmaster.ca/mdprog

  University of Ottawa
  Faculty of Medicine
  Room 2045, 451 Smyth Road
  Ottawa, Ontario
  Canada K1H 8M5
  (613) 562-5409
  E-mail: admissmd@uottowa.ca
  http://www.uottawa.ca/academic/med

  Queen's University
  Faculty of Medicine
  Admissions Office
  Kingston, Ontario
  Canada K7L 3N6
  (613) 533-2542
  http://meds-ss10.meds.queensu.ca

University of Toronto
Faculty of Medicine
Attention: Admissions Office
Toronto, Ontario
Canada M5S 1A8
(416) 978-2717
E-mail: medicine.admiss@utoronto.ca
http://www.library.utoronto.ca/medicine

University of Western Ontario
Faculty of Medicine and Dentistry
Health Sciences Addition
Admissions Office
Health Sciences Center, Room H-104
London, Ontario
Canada N6A 5C1
(519) 661-3744
E-mail: admissions@med.uwo.ca
http://www.med.uwo.ca

Quebec
Universite Laval
Faculty of Medicine
Secretary, Admission Committee
Ste-Foy, Quebec
Canada G1K 7P4
(418) 656-2131, Ext. 2492
E-mail: admission@fmed.ulaval.ca
http://www.fmed.ulaval.ca [In French only]

McGill University
Faculty of Medicine
Admissions Office
3655 Drummond Street
Montreal, Quebec
Canada H3G 1Y6
(514) 398-3517
http://www.med.mcgill.ca

University of Montreal
Faculty of Medicine
Committee on Admission
P.O. Box 6128, Station Centre-Ville
Montreal, Quebec
Canada H3C 3J7
(514) 343-6265
E-mail: admmed@ere.umontreal.ca
http://medes3.med.umontreal.ca [In French only]

University of Sherbrooke
Faculty of Medicine
Admission Office
Sherbrooke, Quebec
Canada J1H 5N4
(819) 564-5208
E-mail: mmoreau@courrier.usherb.ca
http://www.usherb.ca [In French only]

Saskatchewan

University of Saskatchewan
College of Medicine
Secretary, Admissions
B103 Health Sciences Building
107 Wiggins Road
Saskatoon, Saskatchewan
Canada S7N 5E5
(306) 966-8554
http://www.usask.ca/medicine

13 AMCAS and AACOMAS

Now that you've organized yourself and investigated the medical schools, you're ready to apply. Two main application services make it easy for you to apply to most every school by filling out a single, universal application. Most allopathic schools participate in AMCAS (American Medical College Application Service) and all osteopathic schools participate in AACOMAS (American Association of Colleges of Osteopathic Medicine Application Service). You can obtain this universal application through your school's premedical advising office or by contacting the two services directly:

American Medical College Application Service (AMCAS)
2501 M Street, NW, Lobby-26
Washington, DC 20037-1300
(202) 828-0600
http://www.aamc.org

American Association of Colleges of Osteopathic
Medicine Application Service (AACOMAS)
5550 Friendship Boulevard, Suite 310
Chevy Chase, MD 20815-7231
(301) 968-4100
http://www.aacom.org

• **Not every allopathic school participates in AMCAS.** Some schools have their own independent application (see Table 13.1), usually in search of information not obtained via the standard AMCAS form. Currently, some schools are in the process of accepting AMCAS applications, so the list in Table 13.1 may change. Keep this in mind when you actually apply.

91

TABLE 13.1   Non-AMCAS U.S. Allopathic Schools

Baylor College of Medicine
Brown University
Columbia University
Harvard University
Johns Hopkins University
University of Missouri—Columbia
University of Missouri—Kansas City
New York University
University of North Dakota
University of Rochester
University of Texas—Galveston[a]
University of Texas—Houston[a]
University of Texas—San Antonio[a]
University of Texas—Southwestern[a]
Texas A&M
Texas Tech
Yale University

a. Must apply via the University of Texas System Medical Application Center (see address in this chapter).

• **Texas and Canadian schools.** Texas medical schools and Canadian medical schools do *not* participate in AMCAS. You must apply to each one independently, with its own application. However, two other application services exist, one for University of Texas medical schools, another for Ontario medical schools. But these services do not serve every Texas and Canadian medical school, just the University of Texas and Ontario schools. For more information, contact the schools or the application services directly:

University of Texas System Medical Application Center
702 Colorado, Suite 6.400
Austin, TX 78701
(512) 499-4785
uthschro@admin4.hsc.uth.tmc.edu

Ontario Medical School Application Centre
650 Woodlawn Road West
P.O. Box 1328
West Guelph, Ontario N1H 7P4
(519) 823-1940
omsas@netserv.ouac.on.ca

- **AMCAS versus AMCAS-E.** Currently, there are two forms of applications to medical school—the standard American Medical College Application (AMCAS) and the new Electronic Medical College Application (AMCAS-E). Which is better for you? Neither has any particular advantages with regard to chances of admission. The electronic version, however, may be much easier to complete because it's a prompt-driven adventure. If you're computer literate and have an IBM/Windows platform, this may save you a lot of time. You can download the AMCAS-E software at the AAMC Website (http://www.aamc.org). Otherwise, you'll have to sludge through the traditional AMCAS form. Remember, if you prefer the traditional application, **type** the information on the form, regardless of how neat you think your handwriting is. Note: The Association of American Medical Colleges has recently announced that all applications for the 2002 entering medical school class will only be available in the electronic (AMCA-E) version.

- **Academic transcripts.** You will be required to submit to AMCAS/ AACOMAS the official transcripts from each school you have attended. As with the application itself, don't delay with the transcripts. Transcripts may be accepted as early as March. You may want to wait for that semester's grades to be posted before officially submitting your transcripts. But in any case, there's no reason for you to not have your applications submitted by June 1 with the rest of your application.

14 Writing Your Personal Statement

The application essay may be insignificant or very important depending, yes, on what you write about. Don't make the mistake that most people make and write about something that will get your application thrown into the "reject" pile.

Egregious Error: One faculty member at a prestigious medical school told me the story of his first medical school application. He filled in all the blanks, but when he got to the "personal statement" page, he decided he had nothing in particular to say about himself; his grades and extracurricular activities said enough that he didn't have to waste his time writing an essay. So he left his personal statement blank. That's right, blank. Needless to say, he did not get into medical school that year. Next time around, he wrote an essay.

Obviously, only the rare applicant even thinks of leaving the personal statement blank. But the first question that everyone asks about the application essay is, "What should I write about?" The answer is, "Whatever conveys your personality and character to the admissions committee." Yes, that's a very vague answer, but only such a vague statement can encompass the answer for everyone.

A standard approach would be to write about why you want to be a doctor. This should be easy for everyone. If you can't write this essay off the top of your head, you need to reexamine your career choice. But even the most emotional story about watching grandma die from cancer can fail miserably if it's not written well.

A good strategy for your essay is the **intro-body-conclusion method**—that is, three sections, ideally three paragraphs, that (a) introduce you, (b) explain how you made the journey toward a medical career, and (c) conclude by stating what an excellent physician you'll be. As good politicians always say, you have to first tell the crowd what you're going to say, then say it, then conclude by telling them what you've just said.

Self-Diagnosis Exercise

Part A: Before reading the rest of this chapter, use the information from the Self-Diagnosis Exercise in Chapter 1, Part D, to write a practice personal statement essay focusing on your unique individuality.

Part B: Read the rest of this chapter, then rewrite your personal statement essay using what you've learned from this chapter to improve your effort.

Common Essay Mistakes

Many applicants fall prey to several mistakes when writing the essay, and here are ways to avoid the most common failures.

• **You are not Ernest Hemingway.** It's rumored that Hemingway could sit at his desk with a typewriter and a stack of blank paper, begin typing, and without error produce his next novel. No matter how good a writer you are or think you are, your application essay needs to be slick, precise, and most important, contained. And the way to get to this point is by revision, revision, and revision. No admissions committee wants to read your version of *For Whom The Bell Tolls*.

Write and read your essay at least three times over the course of three days. What you think is unbelievable prose one night may turn out to be sappy doggerel the next. Go over it again and again to make sure that every word is exactly the word you want and that you're not repeating the same point over and over again.

The corollary to this rule is that you need to begin writing your essay long before your application is due. Writing it the night before the deadline is a deadly mistake.

- **You will not catch all your mistakes.** No matter how many times you've gone over your own essay, you'll probably overlook a few errors in spelling, grammar, or style. What seems crystal clear to you may not make any sense at all to someone else.

Have at least two friends read and critique your essay. Have at least one stranger read and critique your essay. And make sure that at least one reviewer is someone without a science background. Why not have your mother read your essay? If your own mother doesn't find it appealing or sensible, who will?

- **Concise = Confident.** Dizzy Gillespie said, "If you can't say it in four bars, you can't say it." There's nothing worse than seeing an essay written in a tiny font that fills the entire page. Unfortunately, this happens a lot, probably stemming from the erroneous premed student belief that more is always better.

Make sure your essay fills only 75% of the page by using 12-point Times font. If you can't state your case with 12-point Times on three-quarters of the space allotted, you need to seriously let go of some baggage. Granted, cutting lines from an essay describing your life's desire is an ego-busting experience, but this humbling ability separates the good writers from the bad.

- **I . . . I . . . I . . . I . . . I.** One common problem in most essays is the use of "I" to begin most every sentence. At best, this is a lack of creativity. At worst, it's egotism gone haywire. Not to belittle any applicant's achievements, but nobody wants to read about how you did this, then did that, then thought this, then thought that.

One rule of thumb is to limit sentences that begin with *I* to one per paragraph. And limit the use of *I* to once per sentence. It may not be easy for you, but this is what separates the conceited (poorly written) essay from the humble (successful) one. Consider this an "I told you so" to those who ever thought that English was an easy major.

- **Flashy = Odd.** Flashy is rarely akin to unique individuality. Instead, it's usually a negative indicator of being odd or unusual. The application essay is not the place to show your creativity. You may hear of some applicants who've drawn pictures or written music scores for their essay. No, no, no. Most likely these applicants are still applying to medical school.

And forego the flashy, cursive, or obnoxious type fonts. Again, this is not the way to separate yourself from the pack. Think of it as wearing a red crushed velvet smoking jacket to your interview (see Chapter 18). You definitely will get noticed, but not the way you'd like.

Stick to a 12-point Times font for your personal statement, and keep it an essay. Let your words do the talking, not your fancy color printer.

- **Don't use abbreviations without writing them out first.** Of course, this may be obvious, but it needs to be reiterated simply because so many premed students tend to envision themselves as part of a medical community that loves acronyms. But remember, the admissions committee is as diverse as you can imagine. Everyone is not part of the same community, and thus, they don't all use the same acronyms. This is where nonscience friends are most valuable when reading your essay: Again, if they can't understand it, don't assume that anyone else will.

Egregious Error: One student wrote his essay about the joys of medicine, which he experienced during his job as an emergency medical technician. Of course, he never wrote "emergency medical technician" in his essay, just "EMT." In addition, he described a few experiences with patients using medical lingo such as "running a code," "her BP was sky high," and "a deadly H/H." The essay was also very long, filling the entire page in a 10-point cursive (!) font.

After reading the essay, I asked the student how many admissions committee members he thought would read his essay. He correctly answered, "About fifteen." Then I asked, "How many of them will be physicians?" He couldn't answer that one.

Fact is, there are just as many, if not more, nonclinical basic science faculty on the admissions committee. In fact, some admissions deans themselves are not practicing physicians. Using clinical physician lingo will, at best, not impress them and, at worst, will turn them off. Besides, if you can't explain what you do in simple terms without jargon, you're not exactly promoting your communication abilities, a quality that patients always appreciate in their doctor.

And of course, don't use any abbreviations without writing them out first, and make the font size reasonable so that it can actually be read easily. Do you want your application to be derailed by a technicality?

---

15 Deadline Dummies

The application deadline is assumed by many to be the last date that they can apply. What most people don't know is that concentrating on the deadline guarantees a rejection. This chapter will indicate why the deadline lulls even the best applicants into a false sense of security.

Egregious Error: My best friend and I wanted to apply as early as possible to medical school. We lived just outside Washington, D.C., and the AMCAS (American Medical College Application Service) application center was located in the Dupont Circle area, which is also populated with excellent restaurants. It was the middle of the summer break, and we decided to have our applications ready so that we could drive into Washington on the morning that applications were first due (June 15 that year). We would hand-deliver our applications and have lunch in Dupont Circle.

We arrived at the AMCAS office around 10:30 a.m. and handed our applications to the lady behind the counter. She stamped our return receipts with the numbers 63 and 64. We couldn't believe it! Sixty-two people had somehow gotten their applications in before we did. Granted, being in the 60s is still early enough for most people, but we immediately tried to figure out how so many people had their applications in before us. We decided that some simply arrived earlier than we did, and others used next-day mail service the day before.

The above may not sound like a typical Egregious Error, but the moral of the story is, if we had really been on the ball, we could've made it to Dupont

99

Circle by breakfast and handed in our applications as soon as the door opened. Or you should realize that there are always many more people on the ball before you, so don't slack off.

Although some may say that a deadline is the last day that applications will be accepted, it's more complex than that. Make note of the **first day** that applications are accepted by AMCAS and AACOMAS (American Association of Colleges of Osteopathic Medicine Application Service) (in 1998, it was June 1). In contrast to a deadline, this first day should be given a name—the "lifeline." Most medical schools have rolling admissions. Thus, if you get your application in on the deadline date, it will be received and placed on the bottom of the large pile of applications. As the admissions committee sorts through the thousands of applications before yours, seats in the class will gradually begin to fill. The person on the top of the applicant pile will have a wide-open class waiting for him or her. The person on the bottom of the pile will have maybe a few spaces left over, perhaps only a few waiting-list slots.

What if the application service doesn't send you the applications in time to make the lifeline? This is a common, and unacceptable, excuse. Two simple things you can do to limit the tardiness imposed by application services are to request your applications early and often and have a sample copy of last year's application so that you can practice completing the forms. That way, when the current year's application arrives, you can easily fill it out fast and send it in. The key is to never let yourself get caught in the tardy trap.

Don't take chances. Have your application complete and submitted on the **first day** that they're accepted by AMCAS and AACOMAS. In fact, if you can't submit your application by hand, send it by guaranteed overnight mail the day before it's due. The longer you wait, the more seats will be taken up by other applicants.

16 "Early D" Tragedy

"Early decision" is one of those things that sounds very attractive and may bring immediate joy to many applicants, but it may result only in regret and remorse later. You won't believe some of the reasons that some students apply "Early D." This chapter will explain Early D's pitfalls and reasons to avoid them.

What is early decision? In Early D, you submit only one application to a single medical school that participates in the program. The admissions committee will make one of three decisions for you:

1. **Accept.** If you are accepted, you must enroll in that school. There are no exceptions.

2. **Defer.** If you are deferred, your application is placed in the standard application pool for that medical school. You are then free to apply to any other medical school.

3. **Reject.** If you are rejected, you have not been admitted to that school. You are then free to apply to any other medical school.

Here are the problems with Early D and why only a very small number of students should even consider the program.

• **You're late!** As explained in Chapter 15, your goal is not just to make the deadline but to make the "lifeline." Decisions on Early D applications are made by October 1. If you are not accepted, you can submit applications to other schools only after that date. Applying after any date in October means that your application is much later than most other applicants'. So unless

101

you're almost sure of an acceptance, the only thing you're guaranteed is a late application to any other school. Bad news.

- **You've made your bed, now sleep in it.** There are occasional instances of poorly led premed students who apply Early D to one school for whatever reason, and they get accepted. Then they realize that they should have picked another school or applied to several in the first place. Can you imagine being forced to enroll in a school that you've decided you don't really like? Remember the first Egregious Error mentioned in Chapter 9? Freedom is why our forefathers fought the British. Don't give it up by enrolling in Early D.

- **What are your chances?** For the 1996 entering class, 1,652 of 2,990 Early D applications were accepted. That may seem like a high percentage, but these were all top-caliber applicants. Early D admissions are given only to students who have excelled academically and otherwise. Simply boasting an affectation for a school while submitting a standard or mediocre application does not hold clout with the Early D committee (see the Egregious Error below).

And besides, if you don't make the cut, all your applications to other schools will be late. That should be incentive enough to forego Early D.

Egregious Error: One admissions dean told me a story of a student who applied to his medical school as an early decision applicant. This student was solid but by no means spectacular—a biology major with a 3.50 GPA, a composite 29 on the MCATs, and (you guessed it) experience in a lab as well as volunteer time in a hospital. The admissions dean admitted he was puzzled: "I flipped through the application over and over again looking for a Nobel Prize or something to tell me that he was qualified for Early Decision." But other than a line in the applicant's essay that indicated his fondness for that particular medical school, there was nothing out of the ordinary. "Nice try," the dean said, "but that's not what Early D is about." So the student's application was deferred from Early D and tossed (late) into the pile of other applicants, to be considered in turn.

- **You're late again!** Let's revisit this issue once again but with a positive spin, because most students don't comprehend the gravity of this dilemma. Let's say that you forego Early D and instead submit your application on June 1.

Your application is placed squarely on top of the huge applicant pile and receives consideration as soon as the admissions committee begins work in the fall. If you've lined up all your ducks in a row, you'll receive an interview in early October, and chances are, you have a good shot at acceptance in late October or early November.

Students who apply Early D and who are not accepted will have their applications considered even after some regular admissions candidates are already admitted. Remember, the person on the top of the regular applicant pile will have a wide-open class waiting for him or her. As the admissions committee sorts through thousands of applications, the Early D's who were not accepted early will fall into the pile as if they were regular applicants—that is, late. Since the Early D's who weren't accepted are now in the pile late as regular applicants, they will be scrambling for the few seats that are left, not the wide-open class available to the applicant sitting atop the entire pile.

Remember, don't take chances. Stay away from Early D unless you have an extreme circumstance that requires you to consider only one school. Instead, complete your application early and submit it on the **first day** that they're accepted. Follow the guidelines in Chapter 15. Now do you see again why the September MCAT and Early D are bad ideas?

17 Secondaries and Recommendation Letters

Secondary Applications

Secondary applications are sometimes more important than the "primary" application. Don't ignore them. A secondary application indicates that you've made the first cut, usually the academic cut. Now the schools are interested in more personal information.

Granted, some schools simply ask you to sign a postcard verifying that you've never been convicted of a felony and send it in with a hefty check, but others may ask you to fill out a questionnaire or ask you to write more essays.

Now that you've made the cut, you're competing with the cream of the application crop at that school. Don't stall. You will not receive an acceptance letter without a completed secondary application. Complete it diligently, and follow all the rules for a primary application (send it in early, make no grammatical errors, etc.).

Recommendation Letters

Schools typically ask you to submit your letters of recommendation along with your secondary application. These letters are an essential part of your complete application. Nobody will write a "bad" recommendation letter. But there are no such things as "good" and "bad" letters, just "right" and "wrong" letters. Read on to understand the difference.

Each college or university has its own system for collecting and distributing recommendation letters. Find out early how your school handles these valuable items. And remember, *it's never too early to begin collecting recommendation letters.*

Since recommendation letters are to be submitted with secondary applications, you must again adhere to the same principle of getting everything ready for submission as early as possible. Because recommendation letters are left to the whim of the writer, you may have to be a bit persistent about deadlines here.

What Medical Schools Look for in Recommendation Letters

The purpose of a recommendation letter is to validate your background. It's as simple as that. Anyone can get a letter from friends or family stating that you are a nice person. Anyone can also hype their extracurricular activities to make them sound more impressive than they really are. What you're looking for are letters that validate your academic accomplishments as well as your outside projects. If you really want to show that you've succeeded in something, a reference letter from someone who's supervised you or guided your project should convince the admissions committee what you've really achieved. The "right" letter is one that fleshes out your application by proving your commitment and ability to academic and nonacademic projects. The "wrong" letter simply states the boring, repetitive, and familiar things in every letter—for example, "hard-working," "performed well," and the like. Here are some helpful hints on getting the "right" recommendation letters.

- **Standard letters should be from college faculty or practicing physicians.** These are the bread-and-butter letters that every applicant should have. At least two of your letters must be from science faculty. A physician's letter of recommendation is never a bad thing to have. In fact, some schools require a reference letter from a practicing physician (sometimes a practicing osteopathic physician). But for the successful applicant, these letters are not enough.

- **Other letters should be from people familiar with your other work.** If you have a unique project or experience that defines part of who you are, you should have a letter of reference from someone who has seen your work. Anyone can say they've completed a project or spent time doing this and that. A reference letter proves that someone watched you do the work (and ideally, watched you do it well).

- **Your premedical adviser should write a letter.** Most colleges and universities have premedical advisers on the faculty or staff. These advisers tend to carry significant weight with medical school admissions committees because they've sent students to these schools every year. Medical schools trust their judgment and often rely on their suggestions when making admissions decisions. Most premedical advisers simply write a cover letter distilling the most pertinent excerpts from all your other letters. Others write individual letters themselves. Either way, you should introduce yourself to your premedical adviser and have him or her write a letter. It may be a required ticket to some medical schools.

- **Have more than three letters available.** Most schools want three letters, two from science faculty and one from a nonscience teacher or extracurricular supervisor. You should never have merely three letters of recommendation. You should try to rack up as many as possible. Why? By having a slew of letters available, you can get a good idea of which ones will be better than others. You'll also have a number of "backup" letters in case one reference doesn't follow through. There's nothing worse than what happened to this student:

Egregious Error: One accomplished applicant had his entire application ready and submitted on June 1. He had exactly (only) three recommendation letters, which were promised to him well before any secondary application deadline. After waiting diligently for months, he still had not received word from any medical school. A few phone calls later, he discovered that one of his three references didn't submit his recommendation letter at all. A sad, but true, story. This student's future was left carelessly in the (late) hands of a single reference. Do not let this happen to you.

- **Set earlier deadlines.** If a recommendation letter is due on a particular date far into the future, tell your references that it's actually due up to a month beforehand. You'll be surprised at how lax many university faculty members can be. Of course, you should be reasonable and leave them at least a few weeks to write the letter. But don't leave things to chance, either. By setting the deadline earlier, you give yourself some breathing room.

- **Do *not* get letters from friends, family, politicians, or preachers.** Even if you've performed substantial, validated work with them, there's always the appearance of nepotism or favoritism in these letters. Also, if your work is legitimate, there should be plenty of other people available to vouch for you.

- **Give up your rights.** Most official recommendation letter forms have a space for
  you to waive your right to see the letter. It is commonly acknowledged that if you
  do *not* waive your right to see that letter, it may not be an honest appraisal by the
  writer. Go ahead and waive your rights. Yes, you'll be curious to read what they've
  written about you, but don't take a chance here. If you're really interested in
  reading the letter, ask the writer for a personal copy. Most will be happy to oblige.
  Either way, by having more than three letters available, you can choose those that
  you think are the best even without reading them.

18 Your Interview

The interview is simply the next important step in a successful application, yet most students tend to approach it with either excess paranoia or carelessness. This chapter will explain how to get out of common interview traps.

Egregious Error: One applicant listed "wine tasting" as an outside interest on his application. The interviewer, a prominent medical school professor who didn't like to waste time, noticed this hobby since he also had an interest in wine tasting. He asked the applicant, "What did you think of the Chilean wines of 1993?" The applicant replied, "They were fine." The doctor gave him a stern look and said, "Son, there were no wines from Chile in 1993. This interview is over."

The interview is an important part of your complete application because it provides the school with an opportunity to meet you face-to-face and assess your "people skills." Schools do give plenty of weight to the interview. One study found a good correlation between a student's admission interview score and medical school performance, especially in the later clinical years (Elam & Johnson, 1992). There are numerous stories of applicants with average or even below-average paper applications who nonetheless received an acceptance letter after performing very well in the interview process. There are just as many stories of applicants with stellar academic credentials who were denied admission because of poor interview performance.

What Medical Schools
Look for in Interviews

Most schools are looking for your personal characteristics in your interview. You've already proven your academic mettle with your transcripts, AMCAS application, and essay. Now you have to back up your credentials with some plain old smiling and handshaking. It should be obvious that you must be yourself, be sincere, and show interest in your interviewer, but be prepared for the types of interview styles and questions you may encounter.

• **Bread and butter.** Some interviewers may ask you the stock questions (you can find examples of these stock questions in any standard interview guide) related to medicine, such as, "Why do you want to be a doctor?" Typically, these questions indicate that the interviewer has been blinded to your application, meaning that he or she hasn't seen it; the entire goal is to size you up as a stranger. Don't be fazed. Just answer the questions.

• **More information.** Some may ask specific questions about your application. These people are intrigued with your activities and comments, maybe by your choice of major or by some of the atypical courses you've taken, and they want to know more about you in that way. Again, just be yourself and answer the questions.

• **Psych-out.** There's the story of one faculty member who, while you're answering a question, picks up a newspaper and begins reading. Is he ignoring you? Who knows? It's probably a test to see if you can handle uncomfortable situations. Just be yourself and keep going. There's really no bad method of responding to this type of interview . . . as long as you don't rip the paper out of his hands and demand attention.

• **Shoot the bull.** Then there's the interviewer who doesn't talk about medicine or your background at all. Instead, he talks about last night's basketball game or what the President did last week. This is an attempt to see if you're a real person outside of your academic activities. Go ahead and oblige him. Bring up topics yourself. Engage in a conversation. Show that you have interests outside the classroom.

Sample Questions to Ask During Your Interview and Visit

Most interviewers will end with the granddaddy of all questions: "Do you have any questions for me?" You should be prepared to have at least a few questions, because this is an opportunity not only to find out more information about the school but also to promote your unique interests. Here are some common questions you should consider asking:

- Describe this school's curricular innovations.
- Describe the school's special programs.
- How flexible is your curriculum?

Each of these questions can be followed up by a simple, "I asked that question because I'm really interested in [insert your particular interest here], and I think your program may give me the opportunity to pursue that interest." A discussion will ensue, adding to the interviewer's impression of you as a unique individual.

You may have the opportunity to speak to students at the school. Most schools let the interviewees speak with students alone so that they can "get the skinny" without fear of faculty retribution. Take advantage of this situation. More questions that you may ask include the following:

- How do your students perform on the Boards?
- How good is the financial aid department here?
- How do graduates fare in the "Match" (the process by which fourth-year medical students are assigned to residency programs)?

Remember, the interview is as much an opportunity to sell yourself as it is an opportunity for you to scout the schools. Take advantage of it in both ways. Otherwise, you may never step foot on that campus again.

Interview Outfits

And finally, this shouldn't need to be explicitly stated (you'd be surprised), but your interview outfit should be a sharp, navy blue or dark gray business suit, with a conservative tie for men and hose with sensible shoes for women. Anything out of the ordinary will simply attract more (negative) attention to yourself. If you're wondering whether your outfit is conservative enough, then it probably isn't. Let your words do the talking, not your clothes.

Reference

Elam, C. L., & Johnson, M. M. S. (1992). Prediction of medical students' academic performances: Does the admission interview help? *Academic Medicine, 67,* S28-S30.

19 Which One?

Now that you've been accepted, what a wonderful question to occupy your time: Which medical school should I attend? For some, the question is automatically answered when only one acceptance arrives in the mail. For others, this question is sometimes not easily answered. Here are some things to consider.

• **Why did you apply to this school in the first place?** Ostensibly, you'll have a rank list of schools, or at least a first choice, avoiding any consternation on this decision. However, simply remembering why you applied to a school in the first place may help you decide if you still want to attend that school.

• **Did your visit and interview reinforce the school's strengths?** When you went for your interview, did the school live up to your expectations? Did the students and faculty seem like the kind of people you'd want to hang out with for four years or more? If you applied for a special program, did the school acknowledge the program as one of its strengths?

• **Did the school acknowledge your unique individuality?** If you have a unique interest or project, make sure your school will allow you to continue your pursuits. There's nothing worse than developing a unique interest, applying somewhere with the intention of continuing or enhancing your interests, and then having a school ignore your individuality. Don't let a school shoehorn you into a prepackaged mold by suffocating your creativity.

113

• **Will you be happy at this school for the next four (or more) years?** Sometimes, you just can't pin it down, but some schools give you a positive vibe and others don't. These innate hunches should never be discounted. They usually portend (accurately) your ability to fit into the school's atmosphere. There's nothing wrong with saying, "I just liked it there" or "It just didn't feel right."

• **Where will I get the best education?** Remember, schools and their reputations are never ranked on the basis of *how well they teach* medical students but, rather, on *how selectively they sort* through applications. Thus, it seems that the name of your medical school is more a badge of honor than a measure of your medical education. Try to look past the apparent prestige of the schools and go for the one where you think you'll obtain the best medical education for your needs and interests.

• **Can I afford this school?** Financial aid is a monumental concern for most medical students. As mentioned in Chapter 11, you should have no trouble securing enough loans to cover your medical school expenses. The key to good financial aid is maximizing grants and scholarships and then finding low-interest loans. Each school has a financial aid office designed to provide you with the best package available. **Contact the financial aid office immediately** after you are admitted to discuss your situation and get a head start on applying for financial aid. The third book in this series, *The Right Price,* offers a number of suggestions for ways to procure financial aid.

• **Other sources of aid.** In addition to traditional sources of financial aid, several programs through the military and Public Health Service offer considerable financial support in exchange for medical service. These are legitimate options for anyone interested in such a career. For more information, contact the offices listed below:

U.S. Air Force
Medical Recruiting Division
HQ USAFRS/RSHM
550 D Street West, Suite 1
Randolph AFB, TX 78150-4527

U.S. Army
Medical Corp Branch, Room 2002
1307 3rd Avenue
Fort Knox, KY 40121-2726
(800) 872-2769

U.S. Navy
P.O. Box 9406
Gaithersburg, MD 20898
(800) 327-6289

National Health Services Corp
Scholarship Program
U.S. Public Health Service
1010 Wayne Avenue, Suite 240
Silver Spring, MD 20910
(800) 638-0824

National Health Services Corps
Loan Repayment Programs
4350 East-West Highway, 10th Floor
Bethesda, MD 20814
(301) 594-4400 or (301) 594-4981

20 By Association

There are several medical organizations out there that may provide helpful information about medical school, medical education, and being a doctor. Below is a short list of some organizations specifically designed for medical and even premed students. Also included are a few organizations that provide significant opportunities for premed and medical students. You may find your niche in the activities of some of these associations, and their programs may provide you with opportunities for extracurricular projects, research, or commiseration.

Alpha Epsilon Delta
Premedical Honor Society
P.O. Box 40
Crozet, VA 22932-0040
(804) 823-7057

American Medical Association Medical Student Section
515 North State Street
Chicago, IL. 60610
(312) 464-5000
http://www.ama-assn.org/ama/pub/category/0,1120,14,FF.html

American Medical Student Association
1902 Association Drive
Reston, VA 20191
(703) 620-6600
http://www.amsa.org

American Medical Women's Association
801 N. Fairfax St., Suite 400
Alexandria, VA 22314
(703) 838-0500
http://www.amwa-doc.org

Asian Pacific American Medical Student Association
http://www.apamsa.org

Association of American Medical Colleges
Organization of Student Representatives
2450 N Street, NW
Washington, DC 20037-1127
(202) 828-0682
http://www.aamc.org/about/osr

Christian Medical & Dental Society
P.O. Box 7500
Bristol, TN 37621
423-844-1000
http://www.cmds.org

Medical Students for Choice
2041 Bancroft Way, Suite 201
Berkeley, CA 94704
(510) 540-1195
http://www.ms4c.org

Physicians for a National Health Program
332 S. Michigan, Suite 500
Chicago, IL 60604
(312) 554-0382
http://www.pnhp.org

Student National Medical Association
1012 10th Street, NW
Washington, DC 20001
(202) 371-1616
http://www.snma.org/

Student Osteopathic Medical Association
142 E. Ontario Street
Chicago, IL 60611-2864
(800) 237-SOMA
http://www.studentdoctor.com

Student Physicians for Social Responsibility
1101 14th Street, NW
Washington, DC 20005
(202) 898-0150
http://www.psr.org/spsrhome.htm

Section III
Never Give Up

Self-Diagnosis Exercise

If you're not accepted into a medical school, you have several options. Chapter 21 discusses the pros and cons of reapplying to medical school. Chapter 22 suggests other kinds of practice in the field of health care. And Chapter 23 has information about applying to medical schools outside the United States. Use the following questions to focus your thinking about what you want to do next.

1. What motivates me to want to be a doctor?
   - Helping people
   - Love of science
   - The prestige the profession offers
   - The lifestyle the profession offers
   - Religious/spiritual motivation
   - Opportunity to make good money
   - Other
2. What "shoulds" and "oughts" do I hear as I think about this decision?
3. Who will be disappointed if I don't become a doctor? Who am I most afraid of displeasing?
4. What are my fantasies—good and bad—about becoming a doctor? About *not* becoming a doctor?
5. What am I *not* willing to give up?
6. What do I suspect that I need to look at within myself? Am I ready to look?

7. When I think about becoming a doctor, what part of me feels most neglected? Most unheard? Most unknown?

8. When I think about *not* becoming a doctor, what part of me feels most neglected? Most unheard? Most unknown?

9. What do I look forward to when I think about becoming a doctor?

10. What do I dread when I think about becoming a doctor?

21 Should I Try Again?

Well, that all depends. For some, it's not even a question of whether they want to apply again. For others, this is a very tough decision. There is considerable cost associated with applying to medical school again, especially if you decide to take more courses or enroll in an MCAT (Medical College Admissions Test) review course. Here are a few considerations that may help you make this difficult decision.

- **How can your application improve?** Many premed students make the terrible mistake of simply applying a second time without significant improvements in their application. They ignore the fact that if they were rejected the first time, what makes them more attractive candidates one year later? There must be a **substantial** improvement in your new application for the admissions committee to take notice—for example, a significant GPA or MCAT increase, new publications or awards, an unusual job or extracurricular activity, and so on. Don't count on every other applicant becoming less competitive next year. You must take it on yourself to improve your application significantly.

- **Did you follow all the advice in this book?** Often, the process of applying is just as important as the content of your application. If you feel you made several mistakes like the Egregious Errors described in this book, make sure that you rectify them during the next application cycle. There's no point in making the same mistakes twice, especially since you've read this book.

• **Realistically, what are your chances?** Some students have simple faults in their application—typically, the ones mentioned in this book—that can be easily remedied by the next round of applications. For them, reapplying is not a difficult prospect. However, some students with horrendous grades, little social ability, and no knack for humanity still insist on applying to medical school against many people's advice. You must sit yourself down, look in the mirror, and ask yourself if you have a realistic chance of being admitted to medical school. If the prospects look grim, even with significant effort, move on.

Chapters 22 and 23 suggest options for those of you unable to obtain admission into a medical school. Good luck!

22 Hey, Man, I Just Want to Help People

OK, so you've tried several times to get into medical school; you've taken more courses and taken the MCAT as many times as you could stand, but you still didn't get accepted. And you're fed up with the entire application process. Here's a viable option for you.

Try Another Health Care Career

If, as most premed students say, you really are interested in helping people, then you surely wouldn't mind doing it in a career that has all the exciting patient care possibilities but with a bit less prestige. If you're still willing to get your hands dirty taking care of people, there are numerous options for you. The following careers are by no means "easier" than being a physician. Some of them are just as, if not more, rigorous. One of the careers on this list may appeal to you. Give them all a thought. If you really want to help people, these members of the health care team are just as beneficial and crucial to patient care as physicians. Each suggested profession has contact information where you can obtain further information on each career.

Acupuncture
National Certification Commission for Acupuncture and Oriental Medicine
(NCCAOM)
11 Canal Center Plaza, Suite 300
Alexandria, VA 22314
(703) 548-9004
http://www.nccaom.org

Dental Hygiene

American Dental Hygiene Association
444 North Michigan Avenue, Suite 3400
Chicago, IL 60611
(312) 440-8900
http://www.adha.org

Dentistry

American Dental Association (ADA)
211 East Chicago Avenue
Chicago, IL 60611
(312) 440-2500
http://www.ada.org

Emergency Medical Technician

National Association of Emergency Medical Technicians
408 Monroe Street
Clinton, MS 39056
(800) 34-NAEMT
http://www.naemt.org

Naturopathy

American Association of Naturopathic Physicians
601 Valley Street, Suite 105
Seattle, WA 98109
(206) 298-0126
http://www.naturopathic.org

Nurse

American Nurses Association
600 Maryland Avenue, SW, Suite 100 West
Washington, DC 20024
(800) 274-4ANA
http://www.ana.org

Nurse Midwife

American College of Nurse-Midwives
818 Connecticut Avenue, NW, Suite 900
Washington, DC 20006
(202) 728-9860
http://www.midwife.org

Nurse Practitioner
American Academy of Nurse Practitioners
P.O. Box 12846
Austin, TX 78711
(512) 442-4262
http://www.aanp.org

Occupational Therapy
American Occupational Therapy Association
4720 Montgomery LN.
Bethesda, MD 20814-3425
(301) 652-2682
http://www.aota.org

Optometry
American Academy of Optometry
6110 Executive Boulevard, Suite 506
Rockville, MD 20852
(301) 984-1441
http://www.aaopt.org

Pharmacy
American Pharmaceutical Association
2215 Constitution Avenue, NW
Washington, DC 20037-2985
(202) 628-4410
http://www.aphanet.org

Physical Therapy
American Physical Therapy Association
1111 North Fairfax Street
Alexandria, VA 22314
(703) 684-APTA
http://www.apta.org

Physician Assistant
American Academy of Physician Assistants
950 North Washington Street
Alexandria, VA 22314-1552
(703) 836-2272
http://www.aapa.org

Podiatry
American Podiatric Medical Association
9312 Old Georgetown Road
Bethesda, MD 20814-1698
(301) 571-9200
http://www.apma.org

Psychology
American Psychological Association
750 First Street, NE
Washington, DC 20002
(202) 336-5500
http://www.apa.org

Public Health
American Public Health Association
800 I St., NW
Washington, DC 20001-3710
(202) 777-APHA (2742)
http://www.apha.org

Social Work
National Association of Social Workers
750 First Street, NE, Suite 700
Washington, DC 20002-4241
(202) 408-8600
http://www.naswdc.org

Veterinary Medicine (Hey, man, I just want to help animals)
American Veterinary Medical Association
1931 North Meacham Road, Suite 100
Schaumburg, IL 60173
(847) 925-8070
http://www.avma.org

23 Hey, Man, I Just Want to Be a Doctor

OK, maybe the thought of working as a physician assistant is too unbearable for your physician-intended ego. So you've tried several times again, but you still didn't get accepted. Here's another option for you.

If you still want to be an M.D. and are willing to pay a hefty tuition, you may consider an offshore medical school. You may have heard of some of these schools. Chances are, more than a few physicians in your community may have spent some time at one of these schools. Offshore medical schools are by no means equivalent to medical schools in the United States. None of them is accredited by the same governing bodies as U.S. schools. One major reason is that none of them has a teaching hospital for clinical clerkship. That's right, students at these schools may spend their basic science years on a tropical island, but their clinical years are spent at hospitals throughout the United States or in European countries.

What many people don't know about these schools is that their clinical training is performed in U.S. hospitals—typically, alongside U.S. medical students and residents. And because of this caliber of training, many graduates successfully obtain a slot in an accredited U.S. residency program.

One way to think about the prospects of an offshore education is this: If you go to an offshore school and do well in the first two years, you may have a small chance of transferring to a U.S. medical school. If you can't transfer and continue to perform well during your clinical years at an accredited U.S. hospital, you have a good chance at obtaining a U.S. residency. And after that, you're home free. Graduates of U.S. residencies who have passed all three parts of the medical boards are eligible for state medical licenses, regardless of the medical school they attended. Granted, your chances of becoming an

129

attending physician at Harvard are very, very slim. But if you simply want to practice medicine, an offshore medical education may be your ticket.

Remember, these schools are all very expensive, not including the substantial costs of living in a tropical country. But financial aid is available to most U.S. citizens who attend these schools.

Again, research your school before you send in an application. **And think twice. There are significant obstacles for offshore graduates to obtain clinical clerkships and residencies in the United States. Nothing is guaranteed at these schools.**

As a premedical adviser, I have never and will never recommend an offshore medical school as the first choice for any U.S. citizen. Offshore schools, simply because of the many hurdles that their graduates face to practice in the United States, should always be viewed as a second option only after unsuccessful applications to U.S. allopathic and osteopathic medical schools. The listing here of offshore schools does not constitute in any way a formal endorsement or ranking by the author or publisher.

American University of the Caribbean
Medical Education Information Office
901 Ponce de Leon Boulevard, #201
Coral Gables, FL 33134-3036
(305) 446-0600
http://www.aucmed.edu
Located on the island of Montserrat.

Ross University School of Medicine
460 West 34th Street
12th Floor
New York, NY 10001
(212) 279-5500
California: (818) 248-0812
Midwest: (810) 539-9255
Florida: (954)783-5900
E-mail: info@rossmed.edu
http://www.rossmed.edu
Located on the Caribbean island of Dominica.

Saba University School of Medicine
c/o Education Information Consultants, Inc.
P.O. Box 386
Gardner, MA 01440
(800) 825-7754
E-mail: Saba@tiac.net
http://www.saba.org
Located on Saba island, Netherlands-Antilles.

Spartan Health Sciences University
School of Medicine
P.O. Box 324
St. Jude Highway
Vieux Fort
St. Lucia, West Indies
(758) 454-6128
http://www.worldpaper.com/WMP/spartan.html
Located on the island of St. Lucia.

St. George's University
c/o North American Correspondent
Medical School Services, Ltd.
One East Main Street
Bay Shore, NY 11706-8839
(800) 899-6337
E-mail: sgu_info@sgu.edu
http://www.sga-stgeorges.org
Located on the island of Grenada.

St. Matthews University
School of Medicine
St. Matthew's University School of Medicine, US Office
1005 West College Blvd.
Niceville, FL 32578
http://www.stmatthews.edu
Located on an island, Ambergris Caye, off Belize.

University of the Health Sciences Antigua
School of Medicine Admissions Office
Downhill Campus
P.O. Box 510
St. John's, Antigua
West Indies
(268) 460-1391
E-mail: fmcp@uhsa.edu.ag
Located in Antigua.

Good luck!

Index

133

About the Author

Paul Jung, M.D., is an internal medicine resident at Case Western Reserve University's MetroHealth Medical Center and Director of the Health Policy Leadership Institute. In addition to health policy work with Citizen Action, he worked on the Clinton Administration Health Care Reform Task Force and in San Francisco and Los Angeles on the California Proposition 186 campaign, before serving as the Legislative Affairs Director for the American Medical Student Association. Jung has been a board member of Physicians for a National Health Program, the American Medical Student Association, and the Asian Pacific American Medical Student Association. He is Chair of the National Consortium of Resident Organizations, received the 1998 Fitzhugh Mullan, M.D. Award for Outstanding Resident Physician Leadership, and sits on the American College of Physicians' Council of Associates. He is scheduled to start as a Robert Wood Johnson Clinical Scholar at the Johns Hopkins University School of Medicine in July 2000. Jung has been advising premedical students for several years.